NOT ONE, NOT EVEN ONE

A Memoir of Life-altering Experiences
in Sierra Leone, West Africa

NANCY CHRISTINE EDWARDS

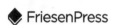 FriesenPress

One Printers Way
Altona, MB R0G 0B0
Canada

www.friesenpress.com

ISBN
978-1-03-913075-3 (Hardcover)
978-1-03-913074-6 (Paperback)
978-1-03-913076-0 (eBook)

1. BIOGRAPHY & AUTOBIOGRAPHY, PERSONAL MEMOIRS

Distributed to the trade by The Ingram Book Company

TABLE OF CONTENTS

Acronyms

BCG	Bacille Calmette-Guérin
CIDA	Canadian International Development Agency
CMO	Chief Medical Officer
CUSO	Canadian University Services Overseas
EDCU	Endemic Disease Control Unit
FGM/C	Female genital mutilation/cutting
GTZ	German Agency for Technical Cooperation
IDRC	International Development Research Centre
Le	Leones, the currency of Sierra Leone
MCH aide	Maternal and child health aide
MRC	Medical Research Council (British)
SECHN	State enrolled community health nurse
TB	Tuberculosis
TBA	Traditional birth attendant

Acknowledgements

This memoir has had a long gestation period both in my mind and on paper. Many helped this project become a reality.

I am indebted to Sister Hilary Lyons, who provided a constant source of pivotal mentorship during my years in Sierra Leone and beyond. Many academic colleagues have allowed and enabled me to follow a sometimes unconventional career path with work streams in international development. I thank you for these opportunities.

I thank my parents, Jean and Inglis, who always showed interest in my Sierra Leonean experiences even when they doubted the sanity of my West African job choices. Growing up, my mother was the resident storyteller in our family. She lit a spark for good storytelling at an early age. My mother and my sister Sheila had the foresight to keep the correspondence I sent to them while I was in West Africa.

Thanks go to the talented group of writers in residence at the Rockefeller Foundation's Bellagio Centre in Northern Italy, whom I met in September 2018. This memoir was not the focus of my residency, but the many genres of writing that other residents shared gave this project momentum.

I thank the Orleans Writing Group, who embraced me and this writing project with enthusiasm. They helped me break free of my academic writing shackles, urging me to add depth and detail to my anecdotes, and to fully insert myself in the stories.

Sister Hilary read an early draft of the memoir. She encouraged me to continue writing. She shared both her published and unpublished writing about her own experiences in the country. Her writings filled some of my knowledge gaps about the long history of service the Holy Rosary Sisters provided in Serabu.

Thanks to my mother and my sister Sheila, who offered helpful reactions to various drafts of chapters. Thanks also to my brother

Brent and his family (Chris, Sydney, and Ryan); to my sister Barbara and her children (Caiden and Kyla); and to my son Andrew and his wife Lauren, who listened to me read selected passages. Lauren brought my photos to life with her expert editing touch (https://rockburn-photography.square.site/).

I thank colleagues and friends, and in particular Lynda, Ken, Connie, Kathy, Barb, Annette, June, Gerry, Nick, Judy, Paul S., Holly, and Peter who read or listened to me read segments of text, providing ongoing encouragement, corrections, and critique. I am grateful for the input of Susan and Yeonjung, who assisted with some of the background research, and Gary, who helped with some fact-checking about Freetown and CUSO.

A shout-out to Merle, a fellow memoirist, who has documented her experiences in Guyana with Cuso International. Merle generously provided tips, suggestions, and encouraging comradery as we each rode the ups and downs of writing.

I especially thank my initial group of beta readers—Susan, Nicki, Sheila, Jean, Elisabeth, Paul T., Phil, and Tom, whose feedback helped me move the memoir to the next level. Jane and Barb read a later version of the manuscript. Your comments propelled me across the finish line.

My biggest vote of thanks goes to my Sierra Leonean teachers, supporters, and assistants. Community health nursing students and the public health staff of Serabu Hospital patiently opened my eyes, helped me bridge cultural divides, and deepened my understanding of Mende ways. To the many traditional birth attendants and maternal and child health aides I met, thank you for sharing your midwifery experiences. Your courage and dedication deeply moved me. To the Endemic Disease Control Unit assistants, who conducted evaluation and research fieldwork under trying conditions, you were a source of inspiration. All of you are unsung public health heroes.

AUTHOR'S NOTES

It has been over three decades since I was last in Sierra Leone. Much has happened since—in the country, in the region, and in my own life. The experiences I recount from Sierra Leone were situated quite early in the country's post-independence period.

I've constructed this memoir from a number of sources. During my first three years in Sierra Leone (1978–1981) as a Canadian University Services Overseas (CUSO) volunteer, I periodically journaled my experiences. I documented more details of my personal and work activities during my last two years in the country (1982–84) when I conducted evaluation and research.

I reviewed documents from Serabu Hospital's archives and reports from Sierra Leone's Ministry of Health, the Bo-Pujehun Rural Development Project, and CUSO/Cuso International. My letters home were another source of information. For the chapter on personal reflections, I relied heavily on publications, official reports, and newspaper articles.

My photos and audio-tapes brought to mind many sights, sounds, and encounters. The book contains some of these photos. Additional pictures are available to peruse on my website (https://www.nancyedwards.ca).

I conferred with colleagues with whom I worked in Sierra Leone. Connie and David, both CUSO volunteers in Serabu, shared anecdotes and documents. In 2019, I had the opportunity to rendezvous with four Holy Rosary Sisters I had worked alongside in Serabu. They rekindled memories and added detail to stories.

When I lived in Sierra Leone, I was able to converse in basic Krio. My understanding of Mende was scant. Colleagues and students provided translation. My journal entries of stories and dialogue in the villages are those English translations. I primarily recreated dialogue from notes in my journals, but some came from memory. I made some adjustments to dialogue to improve the narrative flow.

My first visit to Blama is a composite story, which documents interactions that occurred during several visits to the village. I combined descriptions of context from different villages to add depth to a few stories.

I've used consistent spelling for place names within the memoir but different spellings are used for some communities. For example, Mattru is sometimes spelt with one "t" as shown on the United Nations' map. Serabu was located in Bumpe Ngao Chiefdom but I use the shorter name (Bumpe Chiefdom) in most of the memoir as this was the local term. It is not to be confused with Bumpeh Chiefdom in Moyamba District.

The Sande Society is also referred to by the Sherbro term *Bundu* (also spelt *Bondo*). I use *Bundu* throughout as this was the more common conversational term where I lived. I use the alternate spelling for *Bundu* when quoting a citation with the other spelling. Mende words are written phonetically.

CUSO and Cuso International are mentioned several times. The name change occurred in 1981; I use the organizational name that is historically correct. Common use of the terms less-developed country, third-world country, and low-income country has shifted since the 1970s. I applied the terminology that is most consistent with the different time periods reflected in the memoir. I avoided the term "developing country", as this can be construed as pejorative.

I used pseudonyms for several individuals either to respect their privacy or because I failed to record their names in my journals. For most people, I have provided only first names to protect their identity.

I tried to record events accurately, but all come with the caveat of my intruding Western viewpoint. Undoubtedly, there are conversational nuances I missed or misconstrued. I apologize for anything I misunderstood or incorrectly described. I am responsible for any errors or omissions.

NOT ONE, NOT EVEN ONE

An African Mende village where
   Ngewo (God) gives and takes,
   rain forest provides and threatens,
   farming feeds and starves,
   piken (children) bring lifetimes of promise or sorrow.
And child-bearing is the lifeline to social security.

Nurses, midwives, dispensers, and doctors,
   in barely accessible clinics, health centres, and hospitals,
   promise treatment and services that
   frighten and cost and displace.
Dislocating villagers
   from *morie* men, traditional birth attendants, and ancestors
   who are trusted to heal and protect and appease.

Nurses squat on cane stools,
asking women about reproductive histories
   for precise numbers,
   for robust indicators,
   for efficient measures of public health impact.
Standard questions cut through women's stories
   to the nub,
   of births and deaths and causes and dates and ages.

An elder edges forward.
Deep wrinkles, gnarled fingers, a halting gait;
   Mama is outside our bandwidth of child-bearing years.
Propelled by determination.
Resolute for an interview.
She WILL add her history to public health records.

Mama sits, bold and deliberate.
Eye to eye with this *pomwei* (foreigner), translation begins.
"Mama – How many pregnancies?"
    "Twelve."
"Mama – How many were born alive?"
    Her voice catches,
    "Seven."
My inquiry softens.
"Mama – How many lived to the age of 5?"
    Tears well. Shoulders slump. Memories flood.
    "None," she whispers.
    "Not one child lives, not even one."

Turning away, she chants.
    "Eh deh to God" (It is up to God),
    wrapping herself in fatalism, quelling grief.
My words can't console.
My words can't express.
My words can't talk.
Her story renders my words empty and superfluous.

In emotive silence we clutch hands and hearts;
    women bridging and feeling and connecting,
    across our cultural divide.
Her shared story,
    her only memory-keeper of lost unborns and newborns.
Mama's imparted narrative
    of losses and sorrow and heartbreak and grief and fatalism,
    now seared deep within me.

Decades since this encounter.
I am beholden to this courageous Mende woman
    to amplify her story through worldly connections,
    to impart the despair of her losses,
    to bolster access to safe care,
    to prevent tragic scenarios of "not one, not even one".

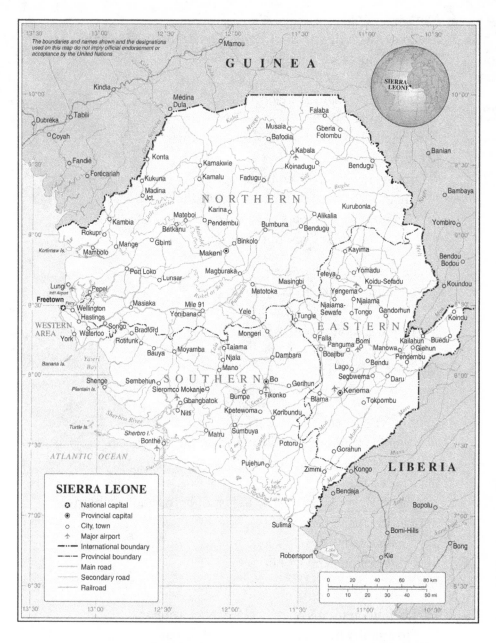

Map of Sierra Leone. Map No. 3902 Rev. 6, September 2014, UNITED NATIONS.

PART 1
STARTING OUT
AUGUST 1978

"What you seek is seeking you." (Rumi)

CHAPTER 1

ARRIVING

I caught my first glimpse of Freetown through the plane window. Mountains near the capital's harbour punched through low storm clouds. In 1462, Pedro de Sintra, the Portuguese explorer who mapped this part of the West African coast, named the area "Serra de Leão"—"Mountains of the Lion". The name stuck, and through the period of British colonization, the country became known as Sierra Leone.

This was neither my first time on the African continent nor my first plunge into a new culture. At the age of 25, this arrival was like no other. I was queasy with excitement and apprehension. I was pining for adventures but starting to doubt whether I was up to the professional and personal challenges that lay ahead. The ache of homesickness was already settling in.

Despite my emotional misgivings, I was certain this was where I was meant to be. Countless discussions and decisions had preceded my trip. I reflected on those as the plane began to descend.

I had cottoned onto the idea of working in a less-developed country in my teens. It started as a vague notion, though its emotive hold ran deep. I couldn't shake it off. Shocking and appalling pictures of Vietnamese children, maimed and orphaned by the war in Vietnam, were often in the news. Their innocent faces and tragic circumstances were riveting, unsettling, and distressing. I wanted to help; I didn't know how.

I had heard about Canadian University Services Overseas (CUSO)[1][2] while I was a student nurse. It was the opportunity I'd been looking for. I attended an information session. I was ready to sign up on graduation, but disappointed to learn that CUSO required nurses to have at least two years of post-graduate clinical experience before being placed overseas. That roadblock gave me pause. There were other pragmatic considerations. Could I tolerate a tropical climate? Could I adapt to living and working in a new culture? Would I enjoy life in an isolated community? I set out to answer those questions, while satisfying my spirit of adventure. I completed a stint as a nurse educator in tropical Townsville, Australia; travelled for eight months through Asia, the Middle East, North Africa, and Europe; and worked as a public health nurse in northern Newfoundland's outports. Four years post-graduation, I confidently answered "yes" to all three questions.

My family was behind my decision to work overseas, sort of. My parents mistook my desire to teach nursing in a third-world country as wanderlust. They tried to dissuade me from signing a CUSO contract during an awkward, long-distance call they initiated while I was living in Newfoundland. In a last-ditch effort, Mum and Dad proposed an alternative to my plans. The Canadian military offered free tuition if I wanted to study to be a medical doctor. They considered this a safer option than venturing to an African nation with CUSO. I was not dissuaded. My decision was final.

I was offered a position in rural Sierra Leone, teaching community health nursing students. I began preparing in earnest. I updated my maternity skills by observing a physician colleague attending deliveries in Baie Verte Hospital. I cracked open my textbook of infectious diseases to read from the pristine pages describing tropical conditions. I attended a leprosy (Hansen's disease) course in Carville, Louisiana and befriended Karen, an American who wanted to work overseas. She worried her career aspirations might not be realized. A family member had been diagnosed with Huntington's chorea; she did not know if she carried the gene. Her preoccupation reinforced my thinking that a couple of years' work in Sierra Leone would be a privilege.

Prepare for Landing

I was jarred back to the flight with the announcement: "Prepare for landing." Suddenly, my new reality was oddly surreal, hugely intimidating, and heavy with responsibility. I was travelling with nine other CUSO volunteers, who would be teaching in secondary schools. I was the only health worker in our group.

Disembarking at Lungi airport, a blast of heat and stifling humidity enveloped me as I walked across the tarmac. I had never felt so alone. Mechanically inching forward in a disorderly line, my international certificate of vaccination was checked, and my passport was stamped. Along with the other volunteers, I was thrust into the frenzy of the arrival's area. CUSO field staff, based in Freetown, helped us navigate the dizzying experience with cryptic instructions.

"Hold onto your passport. Watch for pickpockets. Don't let anyone touch your luggage."

Everything was strangely unfamiliar. This wasn't a temporary tourist destination. This was my new permanent home.

CUSO staff piled our luggage into the back of a mini-bus, as we climbed aboard. Emotions turned inward, all chatter stopped. We were driven into the darkness. The runway lights had been turned off.

Lungi Airport is on a peninsula, which necessitated taking a ferry ride to Freetown. The city's flickering illumination welcomed us, yet the harbour crossing distanced me even further from home. Our bus climbed the steep road up Mount Aureol. As if to reinforce our new reality, rain started pelting down. Torrents of water were pouring off the roof of a Fourah Bay College residence when we arrived. One by one, we were shown to austere and musty rooms. I unpacked the flashlight my father had given me and tucked it under my pillow.

Orientation

CUSO's orientation had started in Ottawa where I was part of a large group of volunteers heading to West Africa. Most were fresh out of university. The majority had been posted to Nigeria to teach in secondary schools.

I joined the handful of health professionals who had left a few days ahead of other volunteers to spend time in London's training mecca for tropical diseases. We took in short lectures and were introduced to resources available from Teaching Aids at Low Cost. I wandered the aisles of the Wellcome Trust Museum, scrutinizing photos of patients with unrecognizable symptoms and specimen bottles labelled with barely pronounceable tropical disease names. Leishmaniasis, lymphatic filariasis, schistosomiasis, onchocerciasis, and African trypanosomiasis. Each new name upped my doubts about being ready for tropical public health work.

Our two-week orientation in Freetown focused on everyday living. I was gripped by a new urgency to absorb all I could. Being with the other volunteers offered me the temporary protection of a social cocoon. CUSO staff answered our barrage of questions. I struggled through language lessons in Krio, the lingua franca of Freetown. Some phrases were fun and easy to learn since they were peppered with English words: "*Morning-oh*" (Good Morning); "*How di body?*" (How are you?); "*Belly done full bad-bad one*" (My stomach is full); "*Uh-say you deh go?*" (Where are you going?); and, "*Lessem deh price small-small, do yah*" (Lower the price a little, do so). Other Krio expressions were rich in vocabulary borrowed from Portuguese and Yoruba, a Nigerian language.

Over meals, volunteers chatted about practical matters like how to dry laundry in the dripping humidity; where to buy batteries; the cost of a postage stamp for a letter home; and the necessity of a mosquito net, if any buzz-free sleep was to be had. I reminded others to take their anti-malarials. We swapped gecko, cockroach, and spider stories. I tried out my new Krio phrases.

Fourah Bay's sprawling campus was quiet; the new semester was not due to begin for a few weeks. When the rain let up, we had a bird's-eye view of the compact city and wide harbour. Life on campus was vaguely familiar; a world away from street-level poverty at the bottom of the mountain.

Short lectures on Sierra Leone's colonial history, post-independence politics and economics, and Creole culture and religion left me with more questions than ever about the country and its peoples. I was rattled by descriptions of Sierra Leone's rich resources (diamonds, gold, bauxite, rutile, and iron ore). The country, with barely three million people, was drowning in poverty and seriously lacked basic infrastructure. I understood less and less.

Our volunteer group was driven around the capital in pick-up vans. We tried not to behave like rubber-necking tourists as we were shown Freetown's landmarks. The massive, centuries-old cotton tree in the centre of town had legendary status. This was where Freetown had been named by freed slaves in 1792. Some of these former slaves had come from the Southern States after joining the Loyalists and seeking better lives. Farmland in Nova Scotia was promised and then denied by the British.[3] This connection of people and place to my mother's home province was all news to me.

Freetown had lots of churches. Those built in the 1800s were dignified in their stature and simplicity. Bell towers and spires set apart the Anglican St. George's Cathedral, the Methodist St. John's Maroon Church, and the Catholic Sacred Heart Cathedral. These older places of worship were historic reminders of both the abolitionist movement and missionary zeal. Freed slaves had crossed different ocean paths to Freetown.

The State House was an impressive structure on Tower Hill. It was the residence and workplace of President Siaka Stevens. I found Sierra Leone's political structure perplexing. The one-party state had elected Members of Parliament. Traditional Paramount Chiefs, who ruled Chiefdoms in the provinces, also sat in the legislature. Most of them were men.

The quaint, run-down City Hotel, with its wrap-around veranda, was made famous by the notorious Graham Greene in his 1948 novel *The Heart of the Matter*. At least I'd heard of him. The newer Paramount Hotel was the tallest building in the city. It was upscale and unaffordable on my volunteer wages. The women's hostel was an inexpensive and safe lodging alternative for short stays in Freetown. I didn't pay any attention to accommodation options for the men in our group.

In the centre of town, old and tightly squeezed wooden boarding houses looked like Caribbean housing cousins. Our CUSO field staff officer lived on Signal Hill Road in a middle-class neighbourhood of pastel-coloured and security-guarded, two-storey, cement-block houses with shuttered windows. The social elite lived on the outskirts of town in gated communities of multi-storey homes with manicured gardens, glass windows, gables, and wide verandas. In Freetown's poorest areas, ramshackle dwellings clung to ravines. Rocks held roofs down during storms. Lean-tos made of scrap boards, rusting panels of zinc pan, and tarps provided minimal shelter for the urban poor.

The old colonial customs building was an architectural treasure. The tall, rust-coloured stone structure with its cathedral windows and long front staircase was situated by Freetown's commercial harbour. The port, one of the deepest in the world, had served the allies well during World War II; another point of interest that had not been in my high-school history books.

Our group was shown edifices I never expected to grace as a volunteer: the British Embassy and the Hill Station Club. And there were scary places to avoid: the main police station and Pademba Road Prison.

I was starting to get my bearings. CUSO staff gave us city maps that were full of British place-names: Wilberforce, Leicester, Wellington, Aberdeen, Dalhousie, Sussex, Goderich, and Waterloo. The country had gained its independence in 1961, but a loud colonial ring remained in the former British protectorate.

Maps in hand, we were sent on a discovery exercise to locate essential services. Weaving around hawkers selling goods on sidewalks, I made my way to the post office and to the cramped quarters of the Immigration Department, where residency visas were issued and renewed. Employees were friendly. Government services were available in English, the official language of the country. Krio was the conversational language I overheard.

I checked out shopping options on the main street. A stationary store sold government school books. The hardware store was a handy-man's candy shop. The pharmacy was lightly stocked with over-the-counter drugs that would have required a prescription back home. Sticker shock in the Lebanese-run grocery store made me realize that imported food bordered on unaffordable.

I wandered past a few health clinics and the main hospital. Dental care was only available in Freetown and provided by Sierra Leone's two dentists. Their private offices were tucked into small, run-down buildings. I dared not imagine the dental equipment they were using. Connaught Hospital was the national adult referral hospital. It teemed with outpatients. The hospital had opened in 1912 and showed its age. I rejected it outright as a place to get my medical care.

I was excited to learn of white-sand beaches outside the city centre, but seashore swimming would have to wait until dry season. Lumley Beach would be an enticing reason to visit the capital.

Kissy Market

I was eager to explore Freetown's big market. As our van approached and the road narrowed, I was shaken by the terse instructions of CUSO staff. "Remove your watches, necklaces, and rings. Put your bags out of arm's reach."

In an instant, our mood shifted from jovial to distrusting. I sensed an uncomfortable us-and-them moment. We were newbie volunteers crammed into the back of a pick-up truck, peering into a pulsing throng of people.

Kissy Market was lively, colourful, noisy, and oh-so-black. I wished for my whiteness to disappear. I wanted to be incognito, to belong. I wasn't in Sierra Leone to be with other volunteers. I was in the country to be with local people. Yet, a few cautionary words had triggered my suspicions, created a sense of divide, and positioned me as the outsider I was. My skin colour ran deep into the vestiges of colonialism.

Our vehicle lurched as the driver pressed through the slow-moving mass of noisy sellers and buyers. We had entered well-ordered chaos, all within touching distance. My curious eyes darted from one merchant stall to another, taking in the colourful palette.

Cheap and basic imported wares were on show alongside local goods. Ragtag, secondhand clothes were heaped on plastic ground sheets. Shoes dangled from laces that were tied to anchoring wires that criss-crossed teetering market stalls. I chuckled at the colourful touques laying limp in the steaming heat. Tin utensils, large iron cooking pots, and Chinese enamelware were stacked on low benches, alongside unwrapped bars of dirt-brown washing soap.

Rust-coloured palm oil stained jerry cans. Pungent fish smells wafted from rows of dried bonga and fresh catches. Flies swarmed. Mounds of rice and red chili peppers left me with no illusion as to the featured ingredients in the local *plassauce* (stew). Fruits and vegetables were abundant. I hoped for a similar range of market foods in Serabu.

Nobody seemed to pay us any notice despite our google-eyed people-watching. Sellers fanned themselves between transactions. Women wove their way along imperceptible paths. They stood erect and dignified, balancing goods on their heads while nestling content babies and toddlers secured on their backs with *lappas* (cloths also worn as skirts). I was struck by the air of self-assurance among buyers and sellers. I surmised that market work provided a respectable lifeline to a meagre income.

Up-Country Travel

The inevitable travel to up-country posts loomed. Our volunteer family was about to be dispersed to our places of employment. We were being fanned out to distant lands. The *small-small* confidence I had gained navigating Freetown seemed irrelevant. Ready-or-not, I was being launched. My professional skills would soon be tested.

CUSO staff eased travel arrangements. They purchased tickets so we could bypass the tangled mass of would-be bus passengers crowding the wicket. Fluent in Krio, our CUSO guides located buses heading in the right direction and chatted with distracted drivers, explaining where each of us was to be let off. I was travelling alone. Had my driver been attentive? Did he know where I was supposed to disembark? Was there a toilet on the bus? How could there be so many uncertainties navigating such simple functions?

I calmed as I took my seat. The helter-skelter disorder of privately owned *poda-podas* (half-ton trucks and vans) in the adjacent lorry park was a new distraction. Passengers bartered for fares and then entered the backs of vehicles, where they squeezed into spaces already bulging with people. Huge loads were heaved on top, growing the height of each *poda-poda* two-fold.

Amusing slogans were displayed prominently above the *poda-podas'* windscreens: "God Is Great", "Black Man Transport", "*Eh Deh to God*", and "Destiny: Without Money No Friend". One slogan resonated with my mood and perspective: "No Condition Is Permanent". I whispered the phrase, a new mantra to sooth and comfort me through the weeks and months ahead.

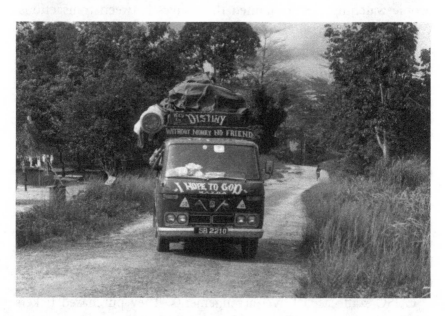

Poda-poda with slogan "Without Money No Friend". The vehicle is being driven on the rough, clay-like gravel of a laterite road.

Without air conditioning, the 150-mile bus ride was hot and sticky. I kept to myself, taking in the rural landscape from my window seat. Subtle landmarks appeared: villages, hills, and junctures in the road.

The rolling countryside had a sameness—thick forest dotted with small patches of cleared land. I saw no barns or silos, no fields of grazing animals, and no tractors or other mechanized farm equipment. My agriculture observations were elementary.

The driver made brief stops in small communities that served as transportation hubs. Hawkers scurried over, hefting basins of food to open bus windows. Passengers thrust payment for *groundnuts* (peanuts), fried plantain, bananas, pineapple, and oranges into vendors' hands. I was too nervous with anticipation to partake.

My fellow travellers' chatter was a labyrinth of tribal languages. The human voices soothed; the foreignness rattled. I would be teaching nurses in English. How would I manage the local Mende language during fieldwork? More disconcerting questions swirled.

Getting to my drop-off village took forever. Before I was ready to disembark, the driver stopped and signalled that he'd reached Serabu Junction, my destination. It looked like every other village we'd already driven through: mud huts with thatched roofs and a few people milling around. There was no roadside snack bar, no taxi stand, no driver waiting to give me a ride. I didn't know how far I was from Serabu. This wasn't the auspicious welcome of which I had dreamed.

A local gestured for me to wait in the shade of a veranda. I felt like a solitary, white-light beacon. When a driver finally showed up, I thought his wrecked car looked like a hostage-taking vehicle. His rapid-fire Krio included one decipherable word "Serabu". I was nervous but all in. The driver stuffed my large suitcase and army-navy surplus rucksack partway into his trunk, strapping them down with thick rubber bands.

I climbed into the cramped back seat and mustered my scant Krio to tell the driver to take me to Serabu Hospital. He needed no explanation. Where else could a *pomwei* with baggage be going? He revved the engine, accentuating its high-pitched whining. The clutch and gear shift ground out of synch as we set off on the rusty-red, laterite clay and gravel road. He dropped me off outside the two-storey convent on the hospital compound.

I was delivered straight into the arms of Sister Hilary Lyons. Years later she remembered my arrival, explaining that visitors to the convent usually asked for Sister Hilary. My first words to her were: "I'm Nancy Edwards."

On hearing my bold greeting, she said to herself, "That's a good one."

Sister Hilary was a remarkable woman, physician, and humanitarian. She would become a dear friend and provide much counsel and mentorship.

CHAPTER 2
PANOPLY OF HEALTH SERVICES

Serabu seemed an unlikely place for an acclaimed hospital and primary health care program. The village was in Bumpe Ngao Chiefdom, one of the larger chiefdoms in the Southern Province and home to just over 30,000. In many ways, Serabu, with its population of approximately 1,700 people, was unremarkable. Farming was the main occupation. Petty traders ran their businesses from veranda stalls. A small food market operated out of the village *barrie* (open-air gazebo-like structure). There was a primary school in Serabu but the closest secondary school was in Bumpe, the Chiefdom's headquarters. The hospital compound was located at one end of the village.

Serabu Hospital began as a small, eight-bed clinic, established by the St. Joseph of Cluny Sisters in 1948. In 1954, another Irish order, the Missionary Sisters of the Holy Rosary, took charge. Sister Hilary Lyons was the principal doctor assigned to the clinic. She came to Sierra Leone from Ireland via a merchant ship in February 1953. The journey had taken nine days. She was 29 years of age, having qualified in medicine eight months before being assigned to the country. I couldn't imagine the weight of responsibilities she had taken on. Describing her wonderment and trepidation on arrival in the country, she wished that the Sisters who met her "would not talk about [work] yet. Anxieties began to bite like a million midges. Would the people accept me? Would I be able to establish any kind of credibility? Would I be able to handle new diseases I had never seen before?"[4]

Sister Hilary's orientation was brief. She did a short stint in Bo, the provincial capital, where the Holy Rosary Sisters rented the Margai

Nursing Home from Dr. Milton Margai, who became the first Prime Minister of independent Sierra Leone in 1961. Sister Hilary was sent to Serabu in October 1954. She explained the circumstances: "The Saint Joseph of Cluny Sisters gave us their house and all that was in it, the clinic, and the school, including the boarding department. They had been much loved in the village of Serabu, which paved the way for our acceptance there."[5]

In the early years, Serabu's medical facilities were ultra-bare-boned. Urgent and desperate cases would arrive at the outpatient clinic doorstep. Sister Hilary was the only doctor in Serabu for nine years. Emergency night surgery was done with the light of bush lamps.

> The clinic [the Sisters] inherited ... was a single building. One part was for delivery of babies, a large room for six to eight cots dressed in European fashion with mosquito nets. There was a large open veranda for clinic. People came in great numbers to avail the services of "*Sista Docta.*" [The small building] was reorganized into a delivery room, a children's ward, a medical ward and behold—using the outpatient room as an improvised theatre we had a kind of operating theatre! It was so elementary ... and yet, I [Sister Hilary] did whatever surgery came my way that was life-saving and learned early on that little is often enough...[6]

Sister Hilary "pressed ahead". In 1956, a separate surgical ward and operating theatre were constructed. In letters to her niece, Sister Hilary reflected on this phase of the work.

> Looking back, I wonder why I started with surgery when my dream was all along wanting that children's ward. The reason seemed to be that emergencies just had to be dealt with. Caesarian sections and strangulated hernias were life-threatening situations. The people liked the drama of surgery. Nothing like

cutting out a problem as a good way of solving one. The Mende liked to see what precisely was removed, tumors or lumps of any description got the highest honours, hernia the most common of conditions was lowly rated, largely because the surgeon had little to show … Once started, other emergencies arrived. A maternity ward followed. The maternity and surgical wards were in separate buildings. They contained eight to twelve beds each.[7]

In the 1950s and 1960s, Serabu was sometimes cut off from Bo, when the hand-drawn ferry stopped working midway along the 33-mile route. Mining companies, doing exploratory geological work in the Southern Province, provided a supply, communication, and transportation life-line for the Sisters. "They did all our messages, groceries, and medicines for a long time."[8]

Two mines—titanium dioxide (rutile) and bauxite—were established later.

On all accounts, the conditions were rudimentary. Sister Hilary became well known for her surgical mastery, her humour, and her boisterous spirit.

Catholicism

Rome was worlds away from Serabu. Nevertheless, Vatican rules and orthodoxy had been very present in the early days of Serabu's medical clinic. Sister Hilary described the attire she initially wore and how this was marginally adapted when she operated on a patient.

In those days I wore, as did we all, an ankle-length gown tied with a leather belt, a scapular, a coiffe (a circular sort of breast plate with a high collar tied at the back). A long Rosary hung from the leather belt. The head gear consisted of an oblong piece of starched linen secured to the head by a cap tied at the back. Over all this went the veil. It was permitted to remove the coiffe for surgery. Over this ensemble went the rubber apron, and in those days, it was heavy rubber. Over all went the sterile gown. As a dress for surgery in the tropics, even if air conditioning had been born [by then], it finally became clear, both to ourselves and our decision makers, that it was nothing short of absurd.[9]

Changes in the Sisters' attire reflected more liberal religious decrees. By the time I landed in Serabu, the Sisters wore plain white uniforms and necklaces with a small metal cross. For Mass and religious celebrations, they wore a simple head cover consisting of a coiffe and veil. Infrequently, the Sisters shared stories of how they had managed clinical emergencies during previously obligatory, monastic periods of grand silence.

Vespers in the convent's small chapel were part of the Sisters' daily practice; a time for collective prayer. The chapel was a single room at the end of the convent. It was stunning in its simplicity. Locally woven country cloths covered the floor and a small altar. Sister Hilary seemed to know when I'd had a particularly difficult work day. She would invite me to join for vespers. The spiritual quiet of the chapel had healing powers. I would leave feeling like I had been wrapped in the soothing comfort of blankets and that my work world would right itself again.

Serabu's Sacred Heart Church was on a small hill, a short walk from the hospital compound. On Sundays, congregational singing wafted through the open-air, upper walls of the church. During my first months in the village, I joined a Peace Corps couple on Friday evenings to play bridge with Paddy Ryan, the parish's Irish priest. My absenteeism at Sunday service never came up in conversation.

Serabu's Primary Health Care Program

By 1970, Serabu Clinic had become a general hospital, with services for surgery, obstetrics, medicine, and pediatrics. Sister Hilary was especially proud of the children's ward where mothers could stay alongside their little ones.

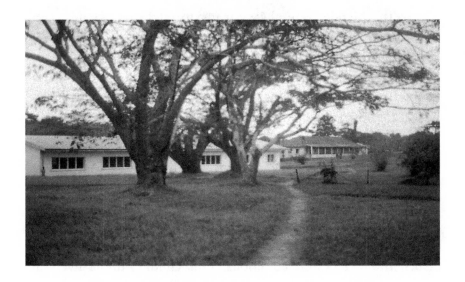

Serabu Hospital grounds. Medical ward is in background and
children's ward is in foreground (circa 1979).

Seven years later, Serabu Hospital had 123 beds, and a staff of five Irish Sisters—three doctors, one registered nurse-midwife, and a nurse educator. All departments had Sierra Leonean staff, most of whom were registered or enrolled nurses. Sierra Leonean nationals were in charge of nursing services, the medical ward, outpatient clinic, pharmacy stores, and laboratory services. Half a dozen volunteer expatriates—physicians, nurses, midwives, and administrators—were on six-month to two-year contracts. Most volunteers were assigned to inpatient services.

Despite these achievements, Sister Hilary had lamented that Serabu Hospital's staff were seeing a troubling revolving door of common, preventable health problems. In 1974, she completed her master's degree at the Institute of Public Health in Antwerp. Sister Hilary described this as an intense experience that equipped her with the skills to bring primary health care to life. It would be co-designed with the Mende people. Sister Hilary explained:

> We tried to find that field (Rumi's) where we could
> dialogue without an agenda. We asked the elders
> of men and women of the main villages to meet us.

The Mende were always ready to talk! They could only meet us at night because they were in their farms during the day as we were in the hospital. The exchanges were profound and sometimes hilarious. This people have wit and wisdom—and soul. In the heart of this people, the individual, the family, the community, and the Secret Societies are united in their quest for health. We found that health was deeper than we had thought. It encompasses the wonder of where God comes into it.[10]

The main thrust of the program was creating an awareness amongst villagers, of their own potential to make health improvements. The targets were ambitious: a) all children under-five years of age immunized; b) adequate nutrition of all under-fives; c) comprehensive antenatal care to all mothers; and d) a reduction in the tuberculosis (TB) defaulter rate and an increase in TB case-finding ability. Care in illness for all community members, improvements in environmental sanitation, and a health education syllabus for school-age children were additional objectives. Mothers and children were priority groups.

Village health committees were a central component of the primary health care program. Members were to be selected by residents of their own villages. Following training, health committees were to help prevent and treat diseases causing the highest morbidity and mortality. They had a liaison function, encouraging villagers to utilize Serabu Hospital when needed. Each person on the committee was responsible to the public health department at Serabu Hospital. Hospital staff were to acknowledge the committee members who referred patients.

The primary health care program was a big vision, filled with possibility. It would have to be phased in. Serabu Hospital received little government funding. Primary health care activities would build on and reinforce existing human resources in the villages.

Launching Stages

The primary health care program was launched in 1975 with a ten-year plan. Stage I (1975–1978) was a pilot. Stage II (1979–1982) would extend activities to section towns in the Chiefdom. Stage III (1982–1985) was envisioned to reach the entire Chiefdom.

The villages of Yengima, Sengima, and Blama, with a total population just under 1,000, were enrolled in the pilot. Between November 1976 and June 1977, detailed baseline data were collected. A physical assessment and simple lab tests were completed for all residents in pilot villages. Health committees were then established and committee members prepared for their roles. An annual reassessment of health status was planned for three consecutive years. Paul Harding, an experienced, state-enrolled nurse was assigned to the village work for the pilot phase. He reported to Sister Hilary. Paul provided training and supportive supervision for the three health committees.

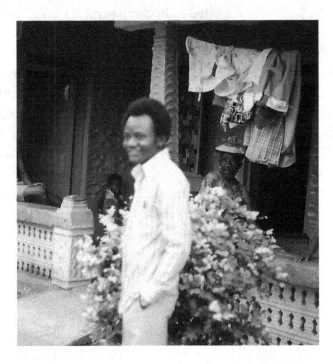

Paul Harding, Serabu Hospital's most experienced public health nurse.

When I arrived in Serabu, the second phase of primary health care was under discussion. Its launch would be boosted by roll-out of the Expanded Program of Immunization in Bumpe Chiefdom. This World Health Organization initiative provided free vaccines for children and tetanus toxoid for women of child-bearing age.

Training Programs

Serabu Hospital had a long history of certificate and on-the-job training. Village maternity assistants had been trained in the 1960s, until that government initiative was phased out. Nurses were trained to assist during surgery, run mobile clinics, and conduct physical assessments. In the mid-1970s, a three-year national State Enrolled Community Health Nurse (SECHN) Program was established in Freetown by the Ministry of Health to replace State Enrolled Nurse training. Staff from Serabu Hospital and Nixon Methodist Memorial Hospital in Segbwema applied to become rural training sites in the Southern and Eastern Provinces, respectively. These approved provincial sites encouraged rural retention of graduates.

Funds for the Serabu-Segbwema Nursing School came from external donors: Misereor (German Catholic Bishops' Organization for Development Cooperation); Cebemo (a Roman Catholic Foundation); and Bread for the World. Like many of Serabu Hospital's programs, external donations were essential for their continued operation.

Training followed an apprenticeship model. Community health students obtained practical experience, while aiding the staff of Serabu's primary health care program. Supervisory responsibilities for students were shared by the public health team and tutors.

Sister Patricia Larkin, a nurse educator who had worked in Nigeria, was in charge of the SECHN program. She ran a tight ship. In addition to her administrative duties, she taught the generic part of the nursing program. Sister Patricia was the eldest among the Sisters, a bit old school in her opinions, and kind rather than stern. She was the only Sister in Serabu who routinely wore her navy-blue, white-rimmed veil.

Government Health Services

Serabu Hospital's services did not operate in a silo. Gradually, the government network of health facilities came into focus for me. Peripheral health units included health centres, treatment centres, and health posts. All were outpatient facilities built and resourced by the government. Health centres were staffed by dispensers, maternal and child health aides (MCH aides), and janitors. Treatment centres were manned by Endemic Disease Control Unit (EDCU) assistants, while maternal and child health posts were run by MCH aides, or occasionally, less qualified village maternity assistants.

Staff had a potpourri of training. Dispensers had completed three years of nursing and an additional 18 months of pharmacy training. EDCU assistants had a patchwork of preparation. When this cadre was first introduced, they were trained for mass communicable disease campaigns. Some were taught how to conduct field surveys. EDCU assistants posted to treatment centres completed several, six-week rotation periods in government hospital departments.

Village maternity assistants had received only three months of training; the program had been discontinued. MCH aides required at least five years of primary school before being accepted into an 18-month training program for mother and child care.

All dispensers, EDCU assistants, and janitors were males; while all MCH aides and village maternity assistants were females. Peripheral health unit staff worked under exacting conditions. I was impressed by their fortitude. Day after day, they provided essential services for local villagers and tackled whatever emergencies arrived at their clinic doors—men with strangulated hernias; farmers with machete injuries, festering wounds, or snakebites; pregnant women with severe anemia or in obstructed labour; and children listless with dehydration, gasping for breath with pneumonia, or convulsing from malaria-induced fever.

Traditional Medicine and Secret Societies

The services of Serabu Hospital and of government-run facilities were situated amidst the work of traditional practitioners, both specialists and generalists. Common to all was the passing of skills and know-how through oral traditions and apprenticeships. Villagers typically sought traditional practitioners before turning to providers trained in Western medicine. The former cadre was trusted, accessible, and affordable. Payment for traditional healers was mainly in kind—rice, chickens, kola nuts, palm wine, or *omolie* (locally brewed gin)—rather than in cash as was required for many of Serabu Hospital's services. Traditional practitioners activated, or not, referrals to the formal health care system.

Traditional birth attendants (TBAs), regardless of age, were also called granny midwives. They were well respected and the most numerous of traditional practitioners. Those who held leadership positions as either a *Sowei* (Head) or *Limba* (Deputy) in the women's *Bundu* Secret Society were revered. *Sowey* were easy to spot as they wore white head ties. TBAs attended most births. Few had any formal training.

I knew nothing of the Secret Societies' pivotal role among the Mende when I arrived in Serabu. Sister Hilary gave me a quick primer. Mende women were not to begin their procreative role until they had been initiated at puberty into the *Bundu* Secret Society. As many as 95% of women in the provinces of Sierra Leone were *Bundu* women. Female circumcision was one of the initiation rites. This information was disquieting. Shivers went up my back.

Boys were initiated into the *Poro* Secret Society. Their initiation rites included circumcision. I never inquired of the age. Discussing *Poro* initiation practices was deemed out-of-bounds for women. *Poro* Society laws discouraged a man from marrying an uninitiated woman.

Taboos and practices of the *Bundu* Secret Society were reinforced by TBAs. Childbearing was women's business. In the villages, women were willing to discuss their pregnancy and postpartum experiences with a male but details of labour and delivery were topics considered strictly off-limits for the opposite sex.

Men were forbidden from entering the cleared area adjacent to a village, where *Bundu* Society initiation rites were performed. Villagers believed that men should and would suffer grave consequences if they witnessed *Bundu* ceremonies. Hernias and hydroceles (fluid-swollen scrotums) could result when men ignored taboos. Similarly, *Poro* Secret Society rites were off-limits for females. Foreigners and other non-members were sternly warned to stay indoors with window shutters closed if either *Poro* or *Bundu* initiation ceremonies were underway.

Some traditional healers, like bone setters and snake-bite healers, focused on physical injuries. Students told me that bamboo splints were woven to hold fractured bones in place, and a chicken leg was broken to gauge healing time. I didn't meet any villagers who had been successfully treated for a poisonous snake bite.

Morie men focused on the social causes and ramifications of illness. They used incantations and traditional herbs that were ingested, rubbed on the skin, or held in protective amulets. Some healers were sought after for their acclaimed treatment of conditions such as TB. *Morie men* were strong social influencers and usually the first to be consulted when someone became ill. They generally stayed clear of Serabu staff during mobile clinics or health committee meetings.

Sorcerers, who were also called *juju* priests, specialized in witchcraft. The arsenal of witches was powerful, their impact could be pervasive. Understanding who caused a person to become ill was a central concern. Sorcerers undid spells so that healing could take place.

While Western-trained health providers in Serabu Hospital understood the importance of traditional consultations, these practices could be extremely frustrating, especially when acutely ill children or labouring women were involved. Consulting meant delays in seeking hospital care, adding to other impediments like getting a patient to hospital, costs of hospital treatment and care, and the need for a household head (husband, father, or uncle) to give permission for hospital admission.

Sometimes patients discharged themselves, or families whisked away hospitalized children against the advice of physicians, seeking traditional healers. These consultations were presumed crucial when patients did not immediately or obviously respond to Western medicine. We never knew if the patient would be brought back to complete their Western treatment.

Traditional medicine was often provided during hospitalization. Children and pregnant women typically had protective amulets tied around their necks, waists, wrists, or ankles. Sister Sheila described making rounds one evening to discover a nurse from the surgical ward providing traditional therapy for a patient; he was moonlighting on the hospital grounds.

Western training left foreigners skeptical if not critical of traditional adjuvant therapy. For the Mende people, Western and traditional medicines were seen as complementary, doubling up the possibility of a good outcome.

The limitations of Western medicine were widely understood. Although injections and surgery were considered more powerful than traditional medicine, village healers and Western-trained practitioners alike knew that Western medicine did not tackle the underlying social causes of patients' illnesses.

A Steep Learning Curve

During my first months in Serabu, I wondered how I would ever traverse the panoply of health services and providers in Bumpe Chiefdom. I felt like a soggy sponge, incapable of taking it all in.

Some components of Serabu Hospital's primary health care program, such as home visits and well-baby clinics, were familiar. However, village health committees, the defining feature of Serabu's approach, were brand new territory for me. I had difficulty unravelling the interplay between Mission Hospital and government services.

Engaging traditional practitioners, whether they be birth atten-dants, *morie men,* or sorcerers, was outside my wheelhouse. I was a neophyte when it came to their community roles and relationships. I had no choice but to confront my biases about their competence. Despite my misgivings, villagers held traditional practitioners in high esteem. They had lineage-earned authority and treatment success stories.

It was hard to wrap my head around the fact that Western treat-ment was judged optional, while traditional treatment was deemed vital. The pertinent question was not choosing between Western and traditional treatment but how to optimize the two in tandem.

Illiteracy was nearly universal; I would have to cross cultural and linguistic barriers I scarcely understood. My well-honed health edu-cation messages were incompatible with local beliefs connected to witchcraft. I would have to navigate social structures like polygamy, Secret Societies, and traditional leadership. I knew next to nothing about these pillars of community strength. My learning curve felt like a steep mountain climb.

Would I ever cease to be a novice? Could I make tangible and meaningful contributions? A few months into my placement, I real-ized that the two-year period for my CUSO contract was much too short a time to have the substantial impact my altruistic-self had dreamed of.

CHAPTER 3
ABUNDANCE OF FIRSTS

Life in Serabu was a massive immersion experience, with many firsts. Work was filled with learning, unlearning, and relearning. Social nuances were hard to grasp. Colleagues answered my tiresome questions, patched over my cultural blunders, and helped me get up to speed as I took on my new responsibilities. Students and staff were patient with my naïveté.

Serabu Hospital's Maternity Ward

My introduction to the hospital began with a tour of the compact maternity ward, a ten-bed unit with an adjacent delivery room. Two rows of iron-frame cots were lined up against the plain walls. Foldable, metal chairs were scattered about.

The small delivery room was at one end of the ward, steps away from the operating theatre. Delivery room equipment was basic— an examining table with stirrups, a rubber ground sheet, a no-frills incubator, forceps, vacuum extractor, vials of oxytocin, glass syringes, an intravenous pole, bottles of saline, and an oxygen tank. A stretcher, two poles threaded through a canvas hammock, was at the ready in a corner.

Grandmothers, sisters, and aunties had accompanied women to the hospital and now doted on them. I sensed an unspoken collective spirit; patients and relatives united through their temporary dislocation from home.

Breastfeeding was the norm. Mothers showed no hint of embarrassment at their bared breasts. Curtains hung between beds, but they were not drawn. One patient's business was everyone's business.

Grannies guided first-time mothers, bringing babies' mouths to nipples, watching infants' rooting reflexes take over. During their hospital stay, family members cooked for patients, washed bed sheets, and provided personal care. Staff concentrated on midwifery responsibilities: clinical assessments and health teaching, monitoring labour, delivering babies, and administering medications.

Wee newborns were swaddled and oblivious to the heat. Their birth skin colour was lighter than their mothers', their eyes more blue than brown. It would be weeks before melanin turned babies' ginger-coloured skin dark and irises a deep chocolate brown. Each precious bundle would be given a name during the traditional naming ceremony that marked an infant surviving its first week of life.

Mothers bathed in the after-glow of birthing. Most were high risk. I was startled by details of women's medical and obstetrical conditions: severe anemia brought on by sickle cell disease and malaria, eclampsia, breech and twin deliveries, and obstructed labour.

I inquired of the mother who cried quietly. No baby lay beside her. The nurse-midwife in charge explained that the woman had been in labour for two days before coming to the hospital from her distant village. Her infant, delivered by caesarian section, was still-born. The young woman had fared better than four others who had been admitted to the maternity ward with a ruptured uterus in the previous year. I had read about a ruptured uterus in an obstetrics book, where it was described as a complication of pregnancy that was almost never seen in a well-functioning health-care system.

It occurred to me that hospital staff saved the lives of women and babies one by one. The primary health care program held the possibility of saving the lives of women and babies village by village.

Blama

We were off to Blama, a small hamlet of 50 or so people and one of the first villages to set up a health committee. I had the nervous jitters and excitement of a child attending their first day of school. Paul was in charge of our visit. I was relying on him to take care of explaining our business in the village and keep me from messing up by prompting me to properly greet the Chief. I would follow his example.

Joseph, a skilled driver, was small in stature and confident in attitude. His touque emphasized his quiet self-assurance. A diligent employee and Serabu Hospital's sole hired driver, Joseph had a mental map of the roads and so-called roads in the Chiefdom. He knew where bush-paths branched off to villages that weren't motorable. He got updates on rainy season road conditions from local *poda-poda* drivers.

Joseph drove the only four-wheel transport owned by the hospital. On occasion, the old van served as a proxy-ambulance. Joseph had helped save lives. I was shown to the front seat, where I sat squished between Joseph and Paul. A crack in the windshield ran through my sight line. The gas gauge needle fluttered on empty. Serabu's petrol delivery was expected the next day or *next tomorrow* (day after tomorrow). I couldn't stop myself and asked if we had enough gas for the trip. Joseph assured me that we had plenty to get to our destination; his tone suggested that I was treading on his domain of expertise. I held off asking my clarifying question: Did he mean enough gas for a one-way or a return trip?

Paul was doing triple duty as my guide, mentor, and translator. He was shy with a gentle laugh. I was awed and intimidated by his extensive public health practice and know-how. Paul had been involved in Serabu's primary health care initiative right from the get-go, spending three weeks out of every four doing village outreach. He was optimistic that village health committees would bring health improvements.

As we were getting to know each other, Paul was sizing me up. This would be my first time meeting committee members. I planned to listen intently and digest whatever unfolded. I hoped to earn a passing grade.

Four student nurses sat on two rows of knee-high wooden benches lining the cargo area of the pick-up van. Joseph tied up the canvas side flaps. It had poured rain during the night, so the road wasn't dusty. We drove out of the hospital compound, taking a quick right onto the narrow road that led out of Serabu. Thick forest lined both sides of the road. The van's springs were well past their prime. When Joseph got the vehicle up to speed, we skimmed over washboard ridges in the laterite road, propelled along like a skipped rock. Our voices turned vibrato.

As we drove through a roadside village, Joseph veered around free-range goats and chickens. Children's voices wafted through the glassless window frames of a two-room mud and wattle primary school. Paul pointed to a native court session; men and women were gathered in the shade of a *barrie*.

Joseph changed gears frequently; the stick shift rubbed against my lower leg. With growing alarm, I realized that Joseph was shifting into low gear to slow the vehicle on undulating hills. Catching my gaze, he explained, *"Brakes no deh work fine."* I made a mental note of that mechanical flaw and watched his technique, because I would be driving students to villages from time to time.

Paul announced our arrival at an inconspicuous bush-path juncture. Joseph had slowed the vehicle by turning off the engine and steering the vehicle as it made pendulum swings between two hills, easing to a stop. We piled out. I was the only one who commented on the stopping exercise.

We were off to talk to the health committee. *"How deh go, deh go?"* (How are things going?). I took the middle position as we walked single file along the narrow and rugged path. I'd been told that the front man spots the snakes and the last in line catches the snakes. I kept my eyes peeled on the shaded ground, watching for critters. Paul instructed me to use a long stride when stepping over a thick pulsing column of soldier ants and then a thin rust-coloured row of stinging fire ants.

Dense forest towered above us. It was mysterious and alive with buzzing insects, bird calls, and monkey chatter. Twittering, chirping, scuffling, and swaying created the unmistakable orchestral music of the jungle. I felt like I was in the heart of Africa.

Too soon, we reached the edge of a large swamp. Its bright shimmer made me squint. Whiffs of decaying matter hung in the humid air. We paused. Paul estimated the water level to be mid-thigh. *A swimmable depth,* I thought. I hauled up my skirt while my male colleagues rolled up their long pants. I concentrated on staying upright in the cool water. Mud squished between my toes. I tried not to imagine lurking creatures, either microscopic or larger. I resumed my precautionary, mid-line position as we waded. I did a quick visual check as we sloshed out of the swamp; everyone looked unscathed. No leeches hung from my legs. I didn't think I'd stepped on any snail shells and reassured myself that the swamp was free of the schistosomiasis vector.

I silently rehearsed my Mende greeting for the Chief as we ducked under the shade of coffee and cacao trees. Paul explained that these cash crops belonged to the Village Chief. Kola nuts were an important symbolic commodity and used during special occasions like infant-naming ceremonies. Joseph had told me that drivers chewed the bitter kola nuts to stay alert.

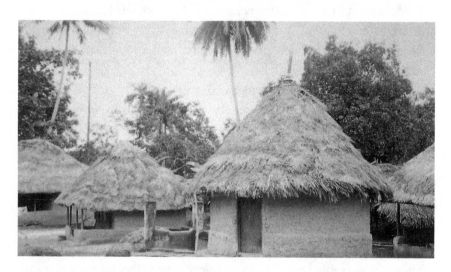

Village of Blama.

The village was more compact than I expected. A small *barrie* was situated near the Chief's home. Mud and wattle homes, daubed with clay, were spaced with only a few feet of bare ground between them. Corrugated zinc pan roofs on a couple of huts were the only hint of wealth. Laundry dried under the protection of verandas. Hand-woven fish nets hung on exterior walls.

Paul tried to keep up with my basic questions.

"What are the clay pots used for?"

"Evaporation from porous pots cools water for drinking. No water treatment is available."

"Why are homes different shapes?"

"Husbands sleep in round huts while wives and *piken* reside in square or rectangular homes."

"What are polygamous family sleeping arrangements?"

"A husband chooses the wife he wants to sleep with on any given night. Breastfeeding women do not have relations with their husbands until infants are weaned."

I needed a crash course on the social and health implications of the polygamous family structure.

Blama's Chief and health committee

We were greeted by the Chief, an older man wearing a brimless, round kufi cap that hugged his head. His ragged shorts drooped on his hips. They were held up by a rope, tied around his lanky waist. His face was etched with furrows. His eyes crinkled as he stepped towards us. He was responsible for welcoming us to the village and giving us permission to speak with health committee members.

Paul showed his respect for the Chief by supporting his right forearm with his left hand as he shook hands, bringing his right hand to his chest to conclude the greeting. I was introduced. Without hesitation, the Chief extended his arm to me; his handshake was hearty and welcoming, his palms rough and calloused from farm work.

Square, shin-high, cane stools were brought for each of us to sit on. After stating the purpose of our visit, Paul invited me to speak. I asked the Chief about their common health problems. Yellow fever and malaria among adults, and malnutrition and diarrhea among *piken* topped the list of ailments. In his side translation for me, Paul clarified that "yellow fever" is the Mende term for jaundice. The direct translation from Mende to English was not enough. Without cultural interpretation, my understanding of a simple Mende message could be distorted.

The conversation veered. The Chief explained that Blama's bigger issue was getting produce to market. They needed a bridge over the swamp so vehicles could reach their village. I was taken aback. I had primed myself for questions like how to prevent malaria and gastro-enteritis. Instead, the Chief dove right into queries about roads and bridges. I bristled. Had my status as a foreigner trumped my role as a nurse? Perhaps he thought I could procure funds for such a project. Haltingly, I stated that funds for such infrastructure were not a real-istic ask for such a small village. Paul must have made adjustments in his translation of my crass statements since the Chief looked neither disappointed nor surprised at my response.

Paul turned to talk of the health committee. The Chief directed us to speak with Isatu, the head TBA, and another woman who had taken on the role of child-care worker. Both were pleased with the lessons they'd been taught. The grannies were called to assist with deliveries in other villages. Isatu explained that the practising TBAs were getting a bit old. She wanted a younger woman to join them to learn their midwifery business.

The child-care worker encouraged women to attend clinic. The distance was a bit far. When mothers went to the dispenser in Taninahun, he did not always have medicine or vaccines. That dis-couraged clinic attendance.

Mansaray

A young woman who looked middle-aged had been hovering off to the side of our talking circle with her four children. After we spoke to the Chief and health committee members, Mansaray inched forward. Her two older children looked to be around four and seven years, and her youngest were twins. They huddled together, all in bare feet. I asked the ages of her children. She was not sure as she had no birth records. She thought her older boy was school age. Since she had no money to pay school fees, her son helped on the farm.

The twins had been born two rainy seasons prior. They looked the size of 12-month-olds. One was perched on her hip; the other was secured to the middle of her back with a *lappa*. Both looked underweight, and the pale colour of their gums and lower eyelids signalled anemia. Paul asked if she had health cards for the twins. She fetched them. Although she could not read, she understood their importance and stored them in their protective plastic wrappers in a large crack in the mud wall above her wood cot. Birth dates entered on the cards indicated the twins were 18 months old. Their immunizations were incomplete; their clinic attendance had dropped off.

One of the twins had signs of kwashiorkor with his swollen feet and sparse, orange-tinted hair. Mansaray explained that her infant son had had several bouts of fever and diarrhea during the rainy season. Mansaray was weaning her babies, and she was concerned.

Paul asked what she fed her twins, explaining that plain rice pap was not enough. He inquired if she grew benniseed, beans, or *groundnuts* on her farm.

With her affirmative reply, Paul encouraged her to add more of these protein sources to the pap, to feed her young twins more frequently, and to avoid putting chili peppers in their food. "Can she bring the twins to clinic for the rest of their immunizations?" I asked.

Mansaray responded hesitantly. "She would try when the farm work was not so busy. Friday clinic was quite far. Her farm was in a different direction. It was difficult to carry both twins to clinic."

Paul turned to me. "Taninahun's clinic is seven miles from Blama."

I gulped. When we encouraged women to get their children immunized, we were asking a lot.

Her older children had extended bellies, probably parasitic worms. The dispenser could give them worm medicine. Shoes might prevent a recurrence of hookworm anemia, but this was an unreasonable suggestion. Paul had focused on the twins. Too much advice could overwhelm.

Departing gift

Flurried activity caught my attention. A young woman was the assigned chicken catcher. She chased the bird, slamming a door as the chicken flew through an entranceway. The race was on. Laughter erupted. The legs of the captured hen were bound together with raffia. All eyes turned to me. I gingerly extended my arms to accept the agitated bird followed by a cumbersome move to dodge its flapping wings. Seeing my startled ineptitude, a student stepped forward to carry the gift. Squawking noises accompanied us on the walk back to the vehicle.

The people of Blama had given me new take-home lessons. I had been struck by their generosity, strength, and self-sufficiency. It was tempting to counter the abundance of health-related problems with a plethora of advice and health education. A one-to-one matching effort was futile. I swallowed hard; advice could harm.

Blama's Chief had identified the pressing problem of market access. I had faltered and too quickly dismissed his request. Paul had filtered and adjusted my responses, keeping me out of trouble. Working as a team had taken on a whole new meaning.

Bumpe Chiefdom's Paramount Chief

All community work involved traditional leaders. Proper protocols had to be followed. Chiefs were key gate-keepers, responsible for the integrity and welfare of their villagers. The strict hierarchy among traditional leaders initially befuddled me. Paramount Chiefs had the overall authority for their Chiefdoms, and resided in their Chiefdom's headquarters. Chiefdoms were divided into sections, each comprised of a section town and many smaller villages.

Bumpe Chiefdom had eleven section towns, each with a Section Chief. Every other community had a Town or Village Chief in accordance with its size. Bumpe was the administrative headquarters. A Paramount Chief, Section Chief, and Town Chief resided there. Navigating their different authorities wasn't straightforward.

Village and Town Chiefs granted visitors permission to stay overnight and gave the go-ahead for activities such as clinics or data collection. A group of elders provided counsel to Chiefs and could be delegated authority for looking after visitors or settling minor disputes. Chiefs' Speakers prepared written communication.

I met our Paramount Chief on my first visit to Bumpe. With a population of 2,100, it was the largest community in the Chiefdom. The town's *barrie* could hold several hundred people. Primary and secondary schools with basic boarding facilities, a busy health centre, and a small and stuffy government office for registering births and deaths were part of Bumpe's infrastructure.

The Paramount Chief's appearance and entourage exuded his authority. He wore a traditional, full-length gown that was generously-embroidered. A dark skull cap, up-turned leather shoes, and a carved, chest-high walking stick completed his outfit. His attendants shuffled behind him with goats in tow. One of the Chief's wives was suffering with advanced-stage breast cancer. She was under the care of Serabu's physician Sisters. We had brought pain medication for her.

Paul introduced me to the Chief and translated as several students looked on. I expressed my sympathy for his wife's condition. We amicably discussed Serabu's primary health care program, and then the Chief gifted me a waist-high, carved wooden statue. I messed up. I politely declined the gift stating it was too generous. Privately, I had no idea where I would put the statue in my small house. Paul interceded, reframing my response to a culturally-appropriate refusal.

The public health team chided my rude behaviour as we rode back to the hospital. I felt sheepish. I should have tempered my Western-informed reactions. Before jumping in, I needed to check the cultural appropriateness of my responses with my co-workers. English to Mende translation could save all of us *pomwei*-provoked embarrassment and missteps.

The Stark Reality of Newborn Tetanus

Our public health team was working an evening shift in Foya, one of the Chiefdom's section towns. Staff and students took their positions in the small open-air *barrie* for the under-five clinic. Each work station was scantily lit by a flickering kerosene bush lamp. Women sat on small benches, cuddling sleepy infants and toddlers. The women too looked tired, having spent the day on their farms. They patiently waited their turn for weight checks, brief health assessments, and immunizations for their children. The night air cooled us.

I was startled by a sudden stirring and plaintive crying. Everyone turned towards the darkness as a woman emerged. She carried an infant and screamed *"soin-soin"* (newborn tetanus). The baby was gripped by convulsions, its head thrown back. As the terrified mother drew closer, I could see the awful telltale signs of tetanus—a clenched jaw, a facial grimace, and rigid arms.

Paul translated. Through mournful sobbing, she breathlessly whispered that she had seen this tetanus before; she had already lost another newborn to this dreaded disease. She was inconsolable. Between sobs, she told us her infant son had been born in the village two weeks prior. He had a strong cry at birth, and he had sucked at her breast until the previous night. She was so afraid he would die. She had no money to go to the hospital. She implored us to save her baby.

Her dilemma was our quandary. Her anguish was our distress. Paul and I quickly conferred. Should we halt the clinic to get the baby to hospital? So many women and children were still waiting for immunizations. Chances for this baby's survival, even with hospital treatment, were slim. Still, we had to explore this option with her. "Does she have her family's permission to take the child to hospital?"

Her downcast eyes told us that she did not. Without permission from her household head, admission to hospital was impossible. "We are so sorry, we have no medicine with us to treat *soin-soin*", Paul explained compassionately. I was too choked up to speak. Without treatment, the infant would not last the night.

I'd heard retrospective accounts of deaths from *soin-soin* in the villages, each told with tearful eyes and a heavy heart. Witnessing this infant in the clutch of tetanus, in the throes of death, and in the loving arms of his devastated mother stirred up a stew of emotions. Grief, frustration, anger, and empathy boiled in my core. How was it that this preventable disease dominated women's fears of their newborns' survival? The loss of this infant to tetanus had to yield more than another deplorable statistic, more than heartbreak for this woman and her family.

As public health workers, we had to pull out full-throttle efforts to prevent the disease, renew attempts to give all pregnant women tetanus toxoid injections, and teach more TBAs to sterilize the instruments used to cut newborns' umbilical cords.

An unusual and stilted silence filled the van as our clinic team headed back to the hospital. Images of the bereft mother trying to comfort her convulsing infant were surely churning and replaying in all of our minds. An innocent newborn victim had fortified our determination to stamp out *soin-soin*.

CHAPTER 4
MORAL DILEMMAS

I had thought my CUSO volunteer status would be a social class equalizer. I wished for my philosophical angst concerning the global injustices of haves and have nots to be quelled. Social class advantages followed me to my post in unexpected ways.

My minority status was multi-pronged. I was white, Anglo-Saxon, and English was my mother tongue. My social advantage turned inside out. To my dismay, my most prominent minority distinction, both perceived and real, was my income bracket. Although I was earning volunteer wages of 240 leones (Le) ($120 Canadian) per month, an amount similar to the wages of my Sierra Leonean nursing colleagues, I was by no means poor. I had the visible trappings of a way-better-than-average salary in Sierra Leone and undeclared wealth in Canada.

I wore prescription glasses and my watch worked. My sandals were made of leather rather than old rubber tire treads, and I had not one, but three pairs of sandals. All my clothes were brand new. I had a flashlight, a tape recorder, and a battery recharger. I played a guitar and owned a camera. I could afford to buy and develop film. An intact mosquito net hung over my bed. I bought rice in the market even when prices sky-rocketed; and I purchased expensive imported foods like milk powder, flour, oatmeal, and golden corn syrup in a grocery store.

It was obvious to my students and Sierra Leonean colleagues that I had been given many opportunities because of my social class. I had flown to Sierra Leone, and I would fly home at the end of my contract. Nobody used the term "white privilege" when speaking to me, though that was the undercurrent.

My students peppered me with questions.

"Have you worked in other countries?"

"Yes, I have worked in Australia and travelled in far-away lands."

"Do you have a husband, a car, a house?"

"No husband but someday I would like to marry. For now, I am a young and single woman. I have owned a car and expect to own another car and a house in the future."

"Do you have dependants like brothers and sisters?"

"I have one brother and two sisters but no dependants. I am not expected to provide financial support for my two younger siblings who are still in school."

The social advantage I had unwittingly brought with me was stirring up new and disquieting self-reflections. Who was going to benefit from my work in Sierra Leone? How could I harness my social class constructively? Was it enough to share my skills and contribute to the education of community health nurses and trainees? Could I do this without displacing Sierra Leoneans or distorting their work? While working in villages, when should I intervene in English? English moments put staff or students into the position of translating for me, taking time away from their primary role and skills as nurses, and disrupting their delivery of health advice.

Everyday life for volunteers was in sharp contrast to everyday life for villagers. This new social gradient added a backdrop of personal unease. How should I allocate my stipend? Could I justify taking a holiday outside the country? I worked hard. I needed a break. I wanted to see more of West Africa. So did my Sierra Leonean colleagues. My financial means made travel a choice.

Was it reasonable for the volunteers at Serabu Hospital to request the hospital van so we could drive to Mokanje mines to enjoy their swimming pool? We rationalized our requests, explaining to the hospital administrator that we did not think our Sierra Leonean colleagues would be interested in swimming, although I don't think we ever asked this question of them. I sensed that Sierra Leonean nationals would not be welcomed by the internationally-owned mining company, which had strictly enforced social and racial class privileges. If we didn't ask Sierra Leonean colleagues to join us, maybe we could keep the lid on that troubling can of worms.

Friday was the designated begging day in our village. If I gave money, food, or clothing to beggars, did this increase their dependency? Would more beggars come to my home with expectations of a hand-out every week? How should I respond when asked to pay primary or secondary school fees for a child? How much should I put aside for this purpose? So many families were in need. Should I hire someone to assist with cooking and cleaning? What was a fair wage for that kind of work?

I had arrived in Serabu, determined to do my own cooking, washing, and house cleaning, not because I did not want to pay for services, but rather because I did not want to enter into a subservient employer-employee relationship. Despite my misgivings, I needed help with chores. Joseph, my first assistant, was bright, shy, and barely a teenager. He rallied his courage to approach me. I agreed to pay his school fees. Joseph used to come on Sunday afternoons. Between the two of us, we'd get the floors of my small home swept and mopped, and my laundry done.

As my classroom and village work increased, and as water shortages became an everyday occurrence, I required more assistance at home. After moving into the village where my roommates and I had no electricity, we hired Foday. He was a hard-working young man who assisted with chores: drawing well water, doing laundry, purchasing market food, and cooking our main meal.

I continued to pay Joseph's school fees; his younger brother, Lawrence, would soon start secondary school. Should I pay school fees for Lawrence? Was I creating social dependence and, if so, was this a good or a bad thing? Would I continue to pay school fees when I left the country and, if so, how could I get funds transferred when his family had no access to banking services? Each question opened another quandary.

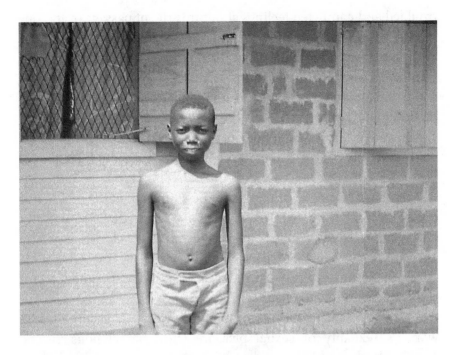

Joseph Campbell standing outside a house on the compound of Serabu Hospital.
Joseph successfully completed secondary school, excelling in language studies. He
obtained a scholarship to study French and planned to attend university. Tragically,
Joseph died shortly after I left the country. May he rest in peace.

Politely, but firmly, my students questioned my motives for working in Sierra Leone. I explained that I wanted to make a positive difference. "But why?" they asked. "Why Serabu where you are working with people you do not know, in a country where you are not a citizen?"

My philosophically-oriented response made no sense to them. Not so different than my failure to provide an adequate answer to similar questions from my family.

Another Kind of Moral Dilemma

Learning of the near-universal *Bundu* Society practice of female circumcision had been a startling revelation. I wrestled with my stance on this practice, as a nurse and a woman. I tried not to disclose my troubled and conflicted feelings about this rite of passage or its consequences through either what I said or how I behaved. Silence was my safe mode. My few brief conversations about female circumcision were with other volunteers or Sister Hilary. I never raised the topic with students or our Sierra Leonean public team. Both groups were predominantly male. I convinced myself that local taboos regarding cross-gender talk of Secret Society practices, and the fact that I was neither Mende nor a member of the *Bundu* Society, put the topics of female and male circumcision off-limits.

After a year in the country, I still knew little about the practice of female circumcision other than a brief anatomical description Sister Hilary provided. It involved partial removal of the clitoris. Bleeding and infections were concerns. Neither Sister Hilary nor nurse-midwives on the maternity ward mentioned obstetrical complications associated with the practice.

I was reluctant to raise the topic of how circumcision affected women's sexuality or sexual pleasure with the religious Sisters. Looking back, sexuality was hardly a word in my own vocabulary. My mother had never sat me down to have "the sex talk".

I never asked my female Mende students to share their personal experiences with initiation rites. None of them divulged information about the initiation period, even when we were in the privacy of the *Bundu* bush. Girls and women took an oath of secrecy when they became members of the *Bundu* Society. I did not press for information, just as I did not take photos of the protected areas for *Bundu* or *Poro* ceremonies on the outskirts of villages. Was this turning a blind eye or showing cultural regard? Maybe I avoided tough but necessary discussions. A communication rift took hold in my mind. I slipped into a culturally-distanced position that kept the topic of *Bundu* initiation rites out-of-bounds.

Conversations about circumcision were sparked among volunteers when the initiates were brought from the *Bundu* bush camp to the village. With their skin coated in a thin layer of smooth white clay, the pubescent initiates were obvious. To me, they looked joyless as they sat quietly and still on verandas. They were on public view as young women. Villagers celebrated their passage into womanhood.

I couldn't imagine the pain these girls must have endured when being cut. Did this recent trauma explain their sullen expressions? I wondered what initiates thought about being marriageable, and whether they had been betrothed to an older man, perhaps someone who already had another wife or wives. Their paths to marriage and becoming mothers had opened up; other life course options had been sealed off.

I wanted to ask initiates more intimate questions. Had they been fearful? How had their anxiety been subdued? What had they been taught about their roles as women, as wives, as mothers? Had they developed stronger bonds with other initiates and their elder mentors? What did they want for their own children? I kept these queries to myself. I tried to honour the *Bundu* Society's oath of secrecy, pushing away my distaste for the act of circumcision.

In brief whispered exchanges with other female volunteers, we debated the potential social consequences of not being initiated. We kept circling back to the practice of circumcision even though we knew there was much more to the initiation period. Initiates were taught dance and song, respect for elders, responsibilities of womanhood, and traditional medicine.

I recollect gossip of a Mende women in our area who had not been circumcised. Reportedly, she was of child-bearing age and unmarried. I don't know if her being single had anything to do with her non-initiation status. Had this marked her as an outcast? The *Bundu* circumcision rite and its social consequences were an enigma.

Female circumcision did not fit into my Western-oriented trichotomy of cultural practices that were harmful, helpful, or harmless. My perspective on female circumcision wavered. Was it unfortunate, unfair, repugnant, or abhorrent? What were the right descriptors? I did not think my Western stance put me in a position to give this practice a definitive label.

I debated my professional obligation to question female circumcision. Should I express my personal opinion? Did I inadvertently signal acceptance of this practice through my silence? As a woman, I was a gender insider; as a non-Mende person, I was a cultural outsider. This moral quagmire was a knotted tangle in my non-confrontational head space.

I kept my silence. Maybe I copped out when I took the easier path of avoidance. I convinced myself that it was better for me to tackle other health issues, wherein I worked respectfully alongside cultural norms of the Mende people.

Rethinking Social Advantage

Tough moral questions did not disappear or become easier to answer with volunteer work. Instead, they took on a new shape and direction. I rethought my ingrained notions of social advantage.

As a foreigner with sideline-observer status of the Mende people, I became aware of social access points I did not have. I was not and would never become a member of the *Bundu* Secret Society. I could neither grasp the full meaning of female circumcision and other initiation practices, nor generate fundamental changes within the *Bundu* Society.

I had no means to obtain or use *halei,* the mysterious medicine of the Mende, which protected in good times and bad. I had no Mende ancestral spirits to ward away harm. I was bereft of proximal immediate family. In Sierra Leone, the only collective to which I vaguely belonged was a motley group of individualistically-oriented volunteers.

I had misconstrued social advantage. Race, income, and education were only superficial indicators. Meaningful social advantage came from the strengths and integrity of social institutions. Throughout their lives, gateways were unlocked for the Mende to grow and be nurtured in the depths of their intergenerational cultural heritage. On these counts, I woefully lacked social advantage.

Volunteerism was not a social equalizer. Nevertheless, being a volunteer deepened my understanding of social integrity and its profound cultural roots. I saw new dimensions of social advantage previously hidden from view.

PART 2
EVERYDAY LIVING

*"If you look too closely at the form,
you'll miss the essence." (Rumi)*

CHAPTER 5
HOUSING AND HOUSEMATES

Daily living was an occasional source of exasperation. The lack of amenities, simple chores, and tangled communication triggered introspection on my Western ways. *"How for do"* (Oh well) was a common refrain. Despite the vexations, my memory banks are filled with shared moments of humour, joy, and poignancy, and the delights of cultural immersion. Plenty of self-effacing experiences still make me chuckle or cringe. I found living in Sierra Leone to be fulfilling, invigorating, and purposeful.

Life in the villages was on full public view. This took some getting used to. Growing up, neighbours had been modestly private. It had been easy to mind your own business. In Serabu, most activities, including those I considered nonpublic, happened outdoors, for all to see, hear, and smell. Food preparation, eating, and breast-feeding; laundering, bathing, and water retrieval; grooming and hair cutting; hammock naps and native court sessions were all done outdoors.

I was drawn to the buzz of daily village work. Groups of women, with babies cradled on their backs, rhythmically pounded food in tall mortars fashioned from tree trunks. Babies dozed through their mothers' labour-intensive chore of food preparation.

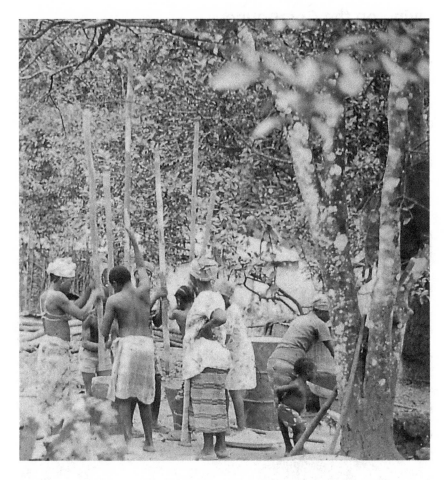

Women pounding food using mortars and pestles.

Three large stones and charred logs defined communal outdoor kitchens. Large iron pots were used to cook rice and *plassauce* in the afternoon; families ate leftover rice in the morning before walking to their farms. Chickens pecked at leftover grains of rice. Nothing went to waste.

My curiosity and intrigue pushed me to poke, stare, and question ways of doing things that were new to me. At times I felt obtrusive, like a rogue anthropologist.

Living on the Compound

I stayed a few months in my first home on the hospital compound, where I lived alone. The house was cozy. I had a bedroom; a small living area with a couple of wooden arm chairs in the centre of the house; and a simple galley kitchen with a few cupboards, a metal countertop, and a basic sink. The house backed onto an orchard of a dozen or so orange and grapefruit trees, with an avocado and breadfruit tree mixed in.

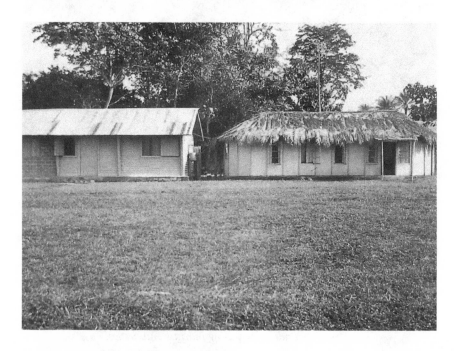

Two homes for volunteers on Serabu Hospital compound. House on the right was my first abode. Both houses had zinc pan roofs. My roof was also covered with palm leaves to reduce the intense heat of the mid-day sun.

The house was connected to the hospital's precarious electrical grid. Two generators provided electricity for the hospital, classrooms, and living quarters during morning and evening hours. The grid powered lights, fridges and fans, the X-ray machine, lab equipment, and the one air conditioner on the hospital compound that was in the operating theatre.

Most of Serabu Hospital's volunteers had shared accommodation. I preferred being on my own. It gave me downtime to process each day's happenings. I turned reflections inward, with no translation required. I played favourite cassette tapes for mood-shifting. Geckos entertained as they went about their business of bug catching.

I had running water because I occupied that house during the rainy season when water levels were high enough in the hospital's shallow well to be pumped through pipes on the compound.

I soon got used to the routine of lights out at 11 PM. In the quiet of the night, sleep came easily. When lights stayed on longer, it usually meant a patient was in the operating theatre for emergency surgery.

The house had an indoor flush toilet for which I was grateful, until one morning when I found a long, shed snakeskin curled around the back of the toilet. I couldn't bring myself to dislodge and discard it, so there it stayed, serving as an anxiety-provoking reminder of intruding reptiles that lived in the area. I had over-estimated how much protection my abode provided. More confirmation of my error in judgment came the day I heard and then saw a couple of rats scurrying overhead in my kitchen. A jolt of fright coursed through me. I had been teaching students about Lassa fever; rats were the vector for this highly fatal disease.

I developed a meticulous, bordering on neurotic, routine for tucking mosquito netting under my mattress. Buzzing insects in my sleeping cocoon were annoying. The image of a snake or rodent gaining entry was terrifying. I intended to stay clear of both. I kept my flashlight with its recharged batteries on the mattress beside me, avoiding the temptation of checking the source of every little sound I heard in the dark. I tried to convince myself that friendly geckos were responsible for the peculiar variety of nighttime noises.

Village House

A few months after arriving in Serabu, the Sisters asked me to move to a larger house they had rented in the village. Despite being kitty-corner from the hospital compound, the house had no electricity.

New volunteers were on their way, and the Sisters wanted me to help them settle in.

My assigned roommates were both nurses. Breege was the youngest. She was a vibrant and playful Irish nurse, who had a mischievous streak. She took to calling herself "Nancy's inmate household pest" because she liked to bait me with her antics.

Dale was a Peace Corps volunteer, with a kind and gentle spirit, and a ready sense of humour. She fit in easily. Dale was a bit of a spectacle in appearance and behaviour. She had strikingly beautiful, long auburn hair. In the late afternoon she'd go for a run. When she reached the end of the paved road in Serabu and was out of village sight, she'd doff her *lappa* and continue running in shorts. Even the volunteers said that her habit of jogging in the heat was off-kilter. Village gossip suggested Dale was possessed by a witch. What else could explain her bizarre behaviour? Dale was hitting her stride supervising student's fieldwork when, after a few months in Serabu, she developed complications related to amebic dysentery and had to be sent home. I missed her company.

By local standards, we occupied a monster home. Our abode was fortress-like, with its cement blocks, corrugated zinc roof, heavy wooden shutters, and barred window frames. We had a veranda, and six rooms; three interior bedrooms and a guest room off the veranda, a common area where we ate and socialized, and a small kitchen for food preparation in the back. Our propane stove was out of commission due to fuel shortages. The backyard was a kitchen extension. That's where Foday cooked dinner over a three-stone fire.

Sister Mary, the hospital administrator, promised to buy a kerosene fridge for our house when one became available in Bo. Kerosene freezers were used to store vaccines in all government health centres. An uninterrupted cold chain is essential to ensure vaccine potency. Staff complained that freezers were finicky, requiring small adjustments to wicks to maintain the right temperature.

The much-anticipated fridge arrived, but it was too big for our single doorways. That left one option. We opened the double doors from my bedroom to the veranda and, by default, my bedroom became its new home. We looked forward to cold drinks and fresh eggs, and frozen meat and chicken to lessen the monotony of dried fish in *plassauce*.

My roommates and I filled up the kerosene canister and lit the small wick. The fridge hummed. In a couple of hours, cold air rushed out when I opened its door. This became a tempting activity since the appliance was a space-heater in my bedroom. I dubbed it our alcoholic fridge because it guzzled kerosene. We tinkered with the pilot light and wick, and adjusted the thermostat to curb its drinking tendencies, all to no avail. Kerosene soon joined the list of fuel sources that were in short supply. While we could make do without a fridge, our kerosene bush lamps were essential. The fridge was transferred to the hospital compound, where it ran on electricity. The nighttime temperature in my bedroom dropped a few degrees.

Our three sources of light failed one evening. We'd run out of kerosene, and there wasn't a drop for purchase in all of Serabu. My flashlight batteries were dead. I had been waiting for the hospital van's next trip to Bo to get a new supply. We had some candles, but we were out of matches and so was the local shopkeeper. I crawled into bed early, feeling annoyed and incompetent. A sense of gratitude slowly took over. I had an intact mosquito net keeping hordes of biting insects at bay. My small inconvenience was no match for the nightly experience of most villagers, who slept without mosquito net protection.

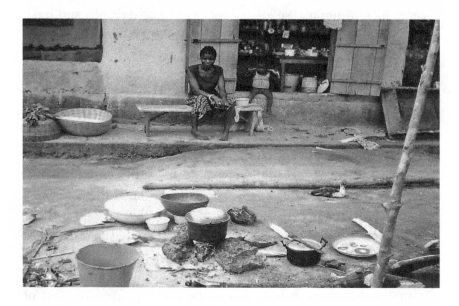

Woman and child sitting in front of small veranda shop in the village of Serabu.
A three-stone cooking fire is in the foreground.

Our low-tech well was in the backyard. A bucket and thick rope sat on a shallow cement apron that protected the well from rainwater runoff. Well water was not potable. Making it so, involved boiling and then filtering water using a charcoal cylinder that fit inside the upper unit of a large metal canister. The contraption sat on our kitchen counter. With the turn of a spigot, we had lukewarm drinking water.

Unlike the well on the hospital compound, our well water did not dramatically recede when the rains stopped because of our proximity to a large mosquito-breeding swamp and a higher groundwater table. Downhill from our well were the adjoined squat latrine and wash yard. Their cement floors were surrounded and divided by a panel of zinc pan. A small opening between the walls and roof let in shafts of light. The latrine had been dug recently, so as outhouses go, it was not very odoriferous.

I assumed the latrine walls offered good protection against reptiles until the night when the faint beam from my flashlight revealed a snake on the floor. I jettisoned myself out of there and moved to the other side of the structure to pee. Other than the slight smell of urine in the wash yard the next morning, proof of my snake encounter was gone.

Our sloping backyard was functional and drab. The area had been fenced with bamboo canes to keep out local goats and chickens. Foday scraped shoots of grass to deter snakes. Our muddy and barren yard was dreary in comparison with the hospital compound, where a gazebo, large shade trees, and flowering plants created a pleasant ambience. In addition to cooking, we used the backyard for private business like shaving our legs, giving each other haircuts, and drying our underwear. Otherwise, the backyard was a lonely place, with few signs of life.

Foday laundered my uniforms, clothes, and bedding. I washed my undies, which provided an unintended source of amusement for patients one sleepy Sunday afternoon. I decided to launder my underwear in the shade near the hospital's well. I think my escapade was mainly about showing off my head-carrying skills. I wrapped my undies in a *lappa* so they would be inconspicuous in the large basket I gauged suitable for a novice headload carrier. I had not practised. Big mistake.

I strutted across the compound to the well. I was in full sight of patients, their families, and hospital staff when my basket fell to the ground near the surgical ward. My underwear spilled out. Possibly sensing my embarrassment, nobody came to assist. I gathered up the evidence and hastened back to my house. Yet another incident suggesting that I lacked basic skills for everyday living.

Nurses kept their uniforms (white dresses for women, white safari jackets and royal blue pants for men) pristine, stain-free, and pressed. I don't know how they did it. Everything was hand-laundered in streams or rivers. Pressing clothes was hot and unpleasant work. Long handles on the heavy metal irons prevented burnt fingers but the hot smouldering charcoal in the iron's belly heated the user like a mini-brazier. Ironing uniforms was not just for esthetics. Tumbu flies lay their eggs on damp clothes laid out to dry. Hatchlings in tainted clothing and underwear burrowed under the wearer's skin and caused painful boils. Ironing killed both eggs and larvae.

At day's end, the front veranda was my go-to place. I'd perch on the half-wall and watch villagers return home from their farms. Men carried light-weight machetes. Women kept pace, despite being laden with loads on their heads and babies or toddlers on their backs. The women's upright posture and steady stride belied their fatigue. Watching them dispelled my tiredness.

I looked forward to seeing a little girl named Fodia. She was three or four years old with the sweetest smile. The first few times I saw her walk by my house, I made eye contact as she clutched her mother's hand. She returned my smile when I waved. One day she asked her mother to stop. Fodia timidly reached for my hand, thereby initiating our regular visits. She giggled when I spoke to her with my rudimentary Mende. In the way that young children do, Fodia uttered Mende phrases expecting me to understand her. I tried to mimic her words and tones, having no clue as to their meaning. Her brief visits were a delight; no expectations and little shared oral language, just tender moments of human connection that made me feel more a part of Serabu's community.

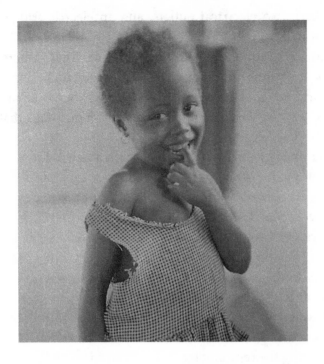

Fodia on one of her evening visits to my home in Serabu village.

Yengima House

Towards the end of my second year, I moved back to the hospital compound where I shared Yengima House with Anne, a newly arrived Peace Corps nurse. The house had been constructed by men from the village of Yengima. Sister Hilary asked them to build a structure using traditional methods and materials. The house had two bedrooms on either side of a common eating and reception area, and an outdoor kitchen. It was complete with wooden shutters, a woven ceiling mat, and a thatched roof of palm fronds. Indoors, the mud and wattle walls had been daubed with white clay.

The house had several deviations from traditional construction. We had a cement floor, screens on the window frames, and a way-bigger-than-average-size latrine. The exterior had been whitewashed with blue-tinted lime. The house had electrical wiring, three light sockets, two electrical outlets, and an electric fridge, but no running water.

We hung a hammock on our back veranda. That's where I practised new Irish tunes for sing-songs on my guitar. Yengima House was remarkably cool even on very hot days. My one substantial complaint was the dust generated by insects in our walls that played havoc with my allergies.

Our outdoor kitchen was equipped with a bench for food preparation and a three-stone fire for cooking. A separate kitchen was good for pest control, warding off the indoor presence of annoying ants and cockroaches that smelled their way to food. Anne and I ate indoors. We kept the legs of our dining table in small cans filled with water, creating tiny moats that made it more difficult for crawling insects to reach food crumbs. We had no desire to add to the hungriest-ants-ever tales that circulated among volunteers.

Foday was still in our employ. He killed a king cobra in the outdoor kitchen one day. I was relieved to have missed the excitement. Ignoring the reproductive capacity of snakes and the potential for small slithering babies, I reassured myself that the cobra had found its way into the kitchen because it was too big to squeeze under the door of our house.

Adjacent to the kitchen was a small wash yard. Six-foot-high palm fronds were held up by bamboo poles, providing ample bathing privacy. When water was plentiful, Foday filled my zinc bucket to the brim and heated it over a three-stone fire. I'd douse myself, scooping up the water with an enamel cup. My daily bath felt luxurious.

When the dry season enveloped us, water shortages were acute. Water for drinking trumped water for bathing. Two cups for bathing and another cup for hair-washing were our self-imposed rations.

Volunteers shared elaborate descriptions of washing techniques. Dr. Carey, a former Peace Corps volunteer, outdid the description of dry-season bathing in a letter he wrote for future medical students coming to Sierra Leone. His description was spot-on, although he claimed that half a bucket of water was needed for his technique. I reckoned we got by with less than half that amount.

With practice in the dry season, you can [bathe] with
half a bucket. To get your armpits rinsed, hold the cup
of water in the ipsilateral hand, flex elbow, and gently
pour water over the shoulder while using contralateral hand with washrag. Throwing cupfuls of water
with the contralateral hand uses too much water.[11]

Our latrine was in a separate hut that was visible from surgical
and maternity wards. Its prominence was like a billboard, providing
a not-so-subtle message to patients that latrines were a good idea.
By village standards, our outhouse was ostentatious. It was circular,
with a cone-shaped thatched roof, ten or so feet in diameter. I had to
crouch to clear the short doorframe.

One evening, as I sauntered into the latrine, I glimpsed a snake
resting beside the wall. I backed away and slammed the door closed.
The intruder had to be dealt with before the outhouse would be
functional. Anne and I were bona fide, snake scaredy-cats. Foday
had gone home for the day, so I ran to the surgical ward pleading
for a couple of male student nurses to kill the critter. The best way to
deal with a snake is to use a long stick, putting as much distance as
possible between you and the reptile. The students' stick was a pole
from the surgical ward's canvas stretcher.

With encouraging cheers from Anne and me, students manoeuvred the pole through the small doorframe, positioning it to clobber
the snake in the cramped space. Shouts and nervous laughter ensued,
but the creature had vanished, escaping the unruly performance.

Not too long after we moved into Yengima House, I bought a
small kitten from the Chief of Masani and named her after her birth-
village. We needed a good rodent catcher since Yengima House
abutted bush and forest. Suspiciously, I never saw or smelled a rodent
carcass. However, I heard enough overhead scuttle to convince me
that Masani was taking her role seriously.

Masani developed a bad habit of peeing in our attic. Since her
rodent-catching space was only separated from our living areas by
a woven mat, this was a problem. Anne was a grandmother with
a calm and compassionate demeanour. Masani peed above her bed

one night, spraying Anne with urine as she fell asleep. With an angry yell, she aggressively called me out. That was the one time I heard Anne swear. I found a new owner for my cat.

Near the Convent

My fourth and final home in Serabu was the old primary boarding school. It had been renovated to accommodate international volunteers. I shared the lodging with Connie, a recently arrived CUSO volunteer who also taught the community health nursing students, and Jo, an Irish volunteer who worked with the hospital administrator. I joked that the Sisters wanted to keep a closer eye on my comings and goings since the new abode was a mere 40 feet from the convent.

Our main floor consisted of a communal living and eating area; an indoor bathroom with a toilet, sink, and shower; and an indoor kitchen with modern conveniences—an electric fridge and gas stove. Running water, a flush toilet, and shower were decadent amenities after my move from Yengima House. We used the partially closed-in veranda as a drying area for laundry during the rainy season. The angle of small, louvered-glass windows on the main floor could be adjusted to catch any breeze. Private bedrooms were on the second floor, including a spare bedroom for visitors.

The hospital received a steady stream of international guests, eager for more details about Serabu's primary health care approach. Visitors spiced up our dinner-time conversations with tidbits of international news and rumours circulating in Freetown.

Guests who stayed longer seemed to be rather eccentric. Possibly we just got to know them better. An international medical student who did an elective at the hospital had been trained as an entomologist. He was intrigued by insects; the dead variety. He was on the hunt for long-horned beetles and pinned his dead, captured insects neatly on a board. It looked like a natural museum display. Cockroaches devoured his entire collection of pinned bugs one night. We were amused by his response to live, flying insects in our unscreened house. He ducked and recoiled, knees to chin, when harmless but annoying sausage flies found their way into our living quarters.

A Peace Corps volunteer, who was posted to another village in Bumpe Chiefdom, stayed with us for a few weeks while she got outpatient treatment. She was the only foreigner in her village and struggled with loneliness and depression. Having recently made the switch to a strict lacto-ovo vegetarian diet, she was preoccupied with sorting out which foods were and were not permitted. I felt sorry for her though I found her singular concentration on food annoying. I soon tired of this topic. Connie and I were supervising students running village clinics. We urged mothers to supplement the diets of their malnourished infants and children with whatever protein foods they had. Whether or not the eggs we got from a hatchery in Walihun were fertilized seemed a trite point of conversation.

CHAPTER 6
SOCIAL SKILLS

Although language acquisition was not my strength, I tried to learn Mende. I hired one of the nursing students as a tutor soon after arriving in Serabu. Twice a week, we reviewed basic vocabulary and practised every-day phrases. Despite my confident start, acquiring even the rudiments of the language proved challenging. My tutor's mother tongue was Mende. English was the language taught in all primary and secondary schools. He had never learned Mende grammar and wrote the language phonetically. Mende speakers were ill-equipped to teach their language.

My tutor and I had no dictionary, no book of easy phrases, and no text of grammatical rules for Mende. Nor did we have written descriptions of the tonal inflections that gave words different meanings. He stressed the importance of tones, demonstrating how subtle, tonal changes to single Mende words modified their meaning. The word for goat also meant water, bring down, and mother-in-law, depending on tonal inflections. He and I concluded that I was tone-deaf. I laughed self-consciously at the misconstrued meaning I introduced into phrases through tonal slips. My tutor wasn't amused.

Language lessons proceeded for weeks; I acquired a few phrases. I could reply when a villager greeted me, alter my greetings to show due regard for a chief, inquire of someone's health, and ask for directions. I had spotty vocabulary for common terms used during clinics. My Mende language acquisition progressed at a snail's pace. My inability to decipher the all-important tones must have exasperated my tutor. He was too polite to say so, but we both knew I was not a model language student.

Social Time

Subtle distinctions separated work time and social time in Serabu. I did not have sufficient Mende or Krio language skills to converse with the locals other than to exchange polite greetings or make simple requests for food or sundry purchases. The public health staff and students translated for me in the villages. I thought it unfair to ask them for after-hours translation services.

Much of my social time was spent with those who had connections to Serabu Hospital. This included volunteers and Sierra Leonean staff, the Sisters, international visitors, and students.

Staff and students supported my acquisition of basic living skills. I was shown how to draw water from a well without wrenching my back, how to use a charcoal iron without burning my fingers or clothes, and how to thoroughly clean a kerosene lamp. I got cooking lessons with local foodstuffs, expanding my *plassauce* repertoire for Sunday dinners when Foday was off. Paul and Simeon taught me how to ride a moped. Students took me to a local farm where I demonstrated how inept I was at using a small knife to harvest rice stalks.

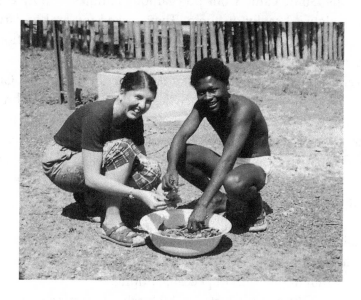

Simeon Tucker giving me plassauce cooking lessons with local foodstuffs in the backyard of my village house in Serabu.

The majority of my students and all of Serabu's Sierra Leonean public health nurses were males. They spent time with my roommates and me on weekends. They usually came unannounced and stayed for an extended period, settling into chairs in our common room. I tried to keep conversations going until I realized our visitors seemed perfectly comfortable with silence. I had trouble deciphering any signals that a visit was coming to a close and guessed it was impolite to suggest time was up. They encouraged us to go about our business while they hung out. They thought we might be lonely.

Our Sierra Leonean colleagues were curious, as was I. Most of my students had had American and British teachers in secondary school. They asked about Canada, my family, my education, and why and how I had come to Sierra Leone. We had wide-ranging exchanges, but avoided the topic of Sierra Leone's politics and never discussed Secret Societies. Shared experiences and stories set us off laughing, either because of surprisingly convergent or wildly divergent perspectives.

Students described their backgrounds, upbringing, villages, and aspirations. Some came from polygamous families. Family expectations weighed heavily on them. They looked forward to earning a salary and providing financial support for the education of younger siblings.

Several students were the sons or daughters of Paramount Chiefs and came from slightly more privileged circumstances. John was one of these. He was gregarious and outgoing. John invited the volunteers to an occasional dance in Serabu; other students were too shy to do so. John was spunky, optimistic, and a bit of a joker, with a wide grin. He was patient and compassionate with mothers and their children.

John was hired as a member of Serabu's public health team when he graduated. So was Thomas, a serious and smart student with strong leadership qualities. Although Thomas looked stern, he had a dry sense of humour with impeccable timing.

Joseph had been a track star in high school, coming second in a national running competition. His promising athletics' career had come to an abrupt end when he broke his femur in an accident. He held no grudges about his misfortune.

Edmund was earnest and rather shy. He came from a small, isolated Sherbro village, near Bonthe. He spoke proudly of his grandmother who had never left her Chiefdom, never ridden in a vehicle, and never seen an airplane. He did not think she'd ever viewed her reflection in a mirror.

Philip was Temne and from the Northern Province. He was a bit of an outsider amongst the predominantly Mende students. Philip was mature and kind. Like some of his classmates, he spoke four languages fluently: English, Krio, his tribal language (Temne), and Mende.

Florence and Alice enjoyed the maternity work. I joined them for a visit with an elderly *Sowei* in Serabu. Their conversation was respectful and engaged. They expressed appreciation for the *Sowei's* long years of midwifery service.

Florence was a go-getter. She had good intuition. I recall a patient Florence brought over to meet us in the tutors' office. The young woman had just been discharged after her initial course of TB treatment; she was heading back to her village. Florence wanted to share the woman's achievement with us to reinforce the importance of the oral medications she would need to take for another year.

Alice wore her emotions on her sleeve. She was usually good-humoured. On our way to a village clinic, her demeanour suddenly changed when we came to a rickety footbridge that had been erected over a swamp by local villagers. Alice was very afraid of drowning. She agreed to cross the bridge by grabbing me around the waist with her eyes shut tightly, as I not-so-confidently guided her across the shaky structure.

I admired the students. Despite humble beginnings, pride in their families and tribal roots was strong. Their immense regard for elders, their collective spirit in the face of difficulties, and their oratorical skills were powerful assets they all had in common.

I found one pattern of behaviour among public health staff and students irksome. An extended family member, often an uncle, would be invoked in a conversation as evidence of a staff or student's good character. This occurred during important exchanges like job interviews or when a special request was being made, such as a leave of absence that required my permission. Normally, these same individuals intimated well-founded confidence in their own abilities.

I would ask myself why they didn't stand on their own two feet when the situation called for it? Years later, a South African colleague taught me the meaning of *Ubuntu*, a Bantu phrase, which translates as: "I am because we are." The penny dropped. I finally understood how important it had been for colleagues to summon others who were influential in their lives into the conversation. My individualistic Western perspective had led me to misconstrue this invocation of family strengths and character as individual weakness. "Mea culpa."

CHAPTER 7

FOOD

I didn't anticipate difficulties adjusting to the tastes or seasonality of local foods. I had an eclectic food palate and enjoyed cooking new dishes. Farm-to-table food was an appealing notion. After experiencing the near-impossibility of growing anything in Newfoundland, I was eager to plant a garden in the tropics.

A Failed Vegetable Garden

I planned a vegetable garden in cahoots with a Peace Corps couple. I was Nancy Reimer's side-kick in the community health office. Her husband, Kevin, assisted with hospital maintenance. We got permission to cultivate a small plot on the hospital compound that was within sight of surgical and maternity wards.

The three of us shared arrogant visions of a demonstration garden. In less megalomaniac moments, Nancy, Kevin, and I relished the anticipated yield of vegetables familiar to our palate. We dreamed of sweet tomatoes rather than bitter jakatoes, and crunchy carrots rather than soggy potato leaves. A self-sufficient approach to gardening was going to get us through the long dry season when market vegetables dwindled.

We purchased simple gardening tools in Bo and hired a man to fence the area to keep out local goats. Sunday mornings, we hoed, planted, weeded, and sweated profusely in the hot sun. Ominously, none of our students commented on the garden. Patients observed us with curiosity from the veranda of the surgical ward. They too offered no commentary. They knew our garden was doomed from the start.

Our plans were impeccable, or so we thought. We planted the garden as the rains subsided. It was near-impossible to imagine what Serabu would be like during the *dries*, but we had planned for the seasonal change. Our plot was approximately 300 feet from the main well for the hospital, easy walking distance to the water source.

As dry season encroached, our plants required daily and then twice-daily watering. The short distance to the well morphed into a long-distance haul as we carried full buckets to our limp plants. Then the acute water shortage, which made hospital operations so formidable, kicked in. Well water on the compound was retrievable in the wee hours of the morning when the groundwater level was higher. We had to line up with other hospital staff who were drawing water essential for day-to-day clinical work. We were in no mood for this competition.

Our determination to harvest fresh vegetables slipped away. The dry season garden failed miserably. It had one redeeming feature. The cassava sticks that our hired help had stuck in the ground as fence posts did take root and provided a crop of edible leaves and tubers for others.

Nancy, Kevin, and I had not even managed to grow a few vegetables. I had a new appreciation for subsistence farmers. Never had I lived so close to the supply end of the food chain. And then I experienced what locals called the hungry season, the period in between depletion of the previous year's harvest and new crop yields. I had cash to buy my way out of food shortages. Farming families did not.

Hungry season lasted for several months, depending on when the rains arrived. The price of rice rose. Fresh produce disappeared from market stalls. My roommates and I asked villagers if they had vegetables to sell. One year, we bought a large yam from an older woman. She had stored it under her bed in the months leading up to the hungry season. I had pangs of guilt. We had left her with cash but deprived her family of food.

What's for Dinner?

Our main meal of the day was rice and a variation of *plassauce*. Foday made the daily market purchases: dried fish, Maggi cubes, palm oil, onions, and seasonal vegetables like potato and cassava greens, pumpkins, and beans. We asked him to go light on the chili peppers. *"Foday, Do yah, do yah, less em small-small."* He did not take our requests seriously. Day by day, Foday added more chili peppers to the *plassauce*, trying to alter our bland palates. Every few weeks he served us a dish that was too fiery hot to eat. We'd reject it as inedible and prepare a dreary backup like oatmeal. The anti-chili-pepper cycle would begin anew. We'd chuckle, knowing that our over-the-top chili pepper meal had been enjoyed by our cook's family or friends.

Palm oil was a main ingredient in *plassauce*. It wasn't long before I sported signs of a vitamin A surplus: an orange hue visible on the palms of my hands and soles of my feet. I developed discerning tastes for *plassauce*. Upland rice smothered with *groundnut* or pumpkin stew were my favourites.

Food Treats

Some food treats required imported ingredients that we shopped for in Bo. With flour, butter, and green mangoes, we baked proxy tart apple pies. I made pseudo-milkshakes from a thick mixture of whole milk powder and water, with ripe banana mashed in. My shakes had the consistency but not the taste of soft ice cream. When eggs were available, the Canadian and European volunteers cooked a communal Sunday brunch special: pancakes slathered with corn syrup.

I satisfied caffeine cravings by scooping finely ground Lebanese coffee into a flask and adding boiling water. A residue settled in our cups. On classroom days, public health tutors touched base with Mr. Reffell, the hospital's nursing director, during morning break. We'd sit in a circle of arm-chairs, swapping updates of hospital happenings and village work. I'd munch my way through handfuls of freshly roasted *groundnuts* that were still covered in their onion-thin parchment.

On weekends, the Sisters often invited the international volunteers who worked at Serabu Hospital for morning tea in their sitting room. Their cook prepared scones, Irish soda bread, and marmalade. What a treat; we tried not to appear greedy.

Delivery of a large flour sack at the baker's small home signalled that fresh loaves of bread might soon be available for purchase. The baker stocked Star beer and pop. On special occasions, like Christmas and Ramadan, he lit his fridge and sold cold drinks. Word got around and Serabu's volunteers met at the makeshift outdoor bar, sitting on wooden stools and exchanging stories while swatting mosquitoes.

As rainy season progressed, fruit returned in abundance. Children clambered up tall mango trees and shook laden branches to urge release of the plump fruit. During citrus season, we enjoyed sliced oranges and grapefruit every night, almost like a dessert.

My favourite thirst-quenching snack was an orange. Women sold them from three-legged stands where the dark green fruit were stacked neatly on enamel trays. The going price was three for five cents, labour included. As customers arrived, women deftly peeled the oily rinds, leaving the thick white albedo intact to hold the juicy pulp. Payment received, the female vendor made a small slice where you sucked the sweet juice, right there, on the spot. With practice, I could squeeze an orange to release every tepid yet refreshing drop, using my teeth to sieve out the pits. Young children quietly sat at their mothers' feet, mastering skills of sorting and stacking fruit, and making change.

Edibles

I extended my list of edible foods, adding potato leaves, okra, jakatoe, pounded cassava leaves, and grated cassava tuber to the edible column of my ledger. Insects remained off-limits. We sifted our flour to remove the weevils.

I was happy to oblige the capture of termites, which arrived with the rains in an orgy of frenzied mating. When I lived in a home with electricity, light bulbs attracted termites in droves. Children rushed in with containers of water, grabbed handfuls of the bugs, drowned them, and removed their wings. They ran home with the dead bodies and women fried their catch. I was told the delicacy was tasty and had a nice crunch. I could not bring myself to try this protein source.

When our public health team held village clinics, women typically cooked rice and *plassauce* that we ate before heading back to Serabu. In the villages, men and older boys ate first; women and young children ate what was left. When our team was served food, there was no gender divide. After washing our hands with water poured from a basin, we'd dig into the communal plate of steaming food usually served on a chipped enamel platter. Sometimes I was given a spoon to eat with. More often I joined colleagues as we used our right hands to form balls of rice with which we scooped up the *plassauce*. The stew was usually made with dried fish, or occasionally with chicken or meat.

All meat was called *bush meat;* that was as much as I wanted to know. I was caught off-guard during a post-clinic gathering with students. We were eating from a common plate of food, chatting about *plassauce* preferences. I veered off script and declared that I had never eaten monkey. I did not disclose that primates were on my non-food list.

"Oh yes, you have eaten monkey," my students chuckled as they responded in a loud chorus to my assertion. Another shift on my edible food ledger.

CHAPTER 8

UP-COUNTRY TRAVEL

Most of my travel involved getting to and from villages in Bumpe Chiefdom. When I travelled to Bo or further afield to the Eastern Province, it was usually in the back of a *poda-poda*. I'd mentally prepare myself for what was sure to be a physically uncomfortable, in-your-face trip. With the command "*Push more, do yah*," the driver's apprentice got passengers to use up every bit of seating space. Bums were pressed together, giving everyone on the hard bench a common height lift when the driver hit road bumps. Layering increased holding capacity. Bare-bottomed babies were passed from one passenger to another, fire-brigade style. Young children sat on the laps of their mothers or other passengers. Chickens with their legs tied together pecked at riders' feet.

Bo had a quaint, small-town ambience. It showed few signs of urban planning. Paved roads ran through the middle of town; some turned into rutted gravel or dirt roads for no obvious rhyme or reason. They reminded me of northern Newfoundland where short sections of road were often paved just before an election; each segment representing an electoral cycle.

Clusters of motley, pastel-coloured shops lined two streets, with living quarters above larger stores. Most shops were owned and run by Lebanese merchants. Some businesses were a front for an elicit diamond trade. Sister Hilary liked to tell her story of uncut diamonds. A Lebanese trader had unwrapped an old hankie to show Mama Hilary the precious crystals he planned to sell on the black market. She did not press for more information.

I asked few questions about diamond mining. Although alluvial mining was active in some of Bumpe Chiefdom's communities, the main areas for diamond mining were in the Eastern province. Diamond trading seemed a distant disconnect from my day-to-day work in farming villages.

The Bank of Sierra Leone had a branch in Bo, but it wasn't practical to open an account. I hid my monthly cash stipend in the locked wardrobe of my bedroom and spent it on food and toiletries; with the balance for hired help, school fees, and social trips to other parts of the country.

Sister Mary's descriptions of lengthy banking procedures affirmed my cash-stashing approach. She had to withdraw funds on staff paydays. The bank issued cash in two-leone notes. Tedious counting of the worn paper currency was repeated in the hospital's administrative office when Sister Mary called in each employee for his/her pay package, noting each transaction in a big ledger.

Bo's general hardware store sold tools and supplies. A stationary store stocked compulsory school books. Street hawkers sold second-hand books, which they laid out on the sidewalk, on top of scruffy sheets of plastic.

A sprawling market was near the shops. Fresh produce and meat, and dried fish filled the air with tell-tale smells. Flies buzzed. Basic goods like soap, cooking utensils, and footwear were available. A small white mosque, with spring-green minarets abutted the market stalls.

Government buildings and services were clustered together. These included the post-office; several Ministry buildings; and the one-storey, sprawling government hospital. I did not step foot in the hospital during my first three years in the country. Occasionally, I spotted a local ambulance delivering supplies like soft drinks, beer, or firewood to homes and cookhouses. I rarely saw an ambulance carrying a patient. I wondered how you even called for an ambulance since nobody had a phone.

A trip to Bo by Serabu Hospital's international staff involved a mandatory check-in at the post office. If the postmaster was present, or an employee knew where the keys were for the mailroom, letters or parcels might be delivered to Serabu when the designated courier returned.

Bo had a light police and military presence. Several rows of over-crowded barracks accommodated these workers and their families at one end of town.

Public schools looked run-down although they were much sturdier and larger than those in most villages. Private schools were scattered around town, reflecting Christian and Muslim groups that had a missionary presence in the country.

Cars and vans that had been donated by bilateral and multilateral aid agencies were the newest, most expensive, and roadworthy vehicles. They outnumbered private cars and taxis. I could piece together sectors, donor countries, and international agencies working in Sierra Leone from the project identifiers stuck on driver and passenger doors. I pondered what messages donor agency vehicles sent to the communities they served.

Bo's garage bustled. It was the central hub for vehicle repairs in the province. Teens and young men hung around, eager to work as informal apprentices, trying to acquire skills for a paying trade. Vehicle repair work was done outdoors. Mango trees and tarps provided shade. Despite the lack of sophisticated equipment, mechanics managed to keep many older vehicles running.

My travels to Bo were for modest reasons. I visited the grocery store for imported staples and made my way to the post office. A few times, I bought colourful *gara* (tie-dye) cloth to sew a new garment. I enjoyed watching tailors who sat in a row of stalls, operating their treadle sewing machines. They copied outfits, cutting the material freehand without using a paper pattern. Their creations were colourful and imaginative.

If I had time for lunch, I'd head to the popular Rio Restaurant. Options listed on the menu over-stated what was available. It was better to ask what *chop* (food) had been cooked that day so I didn't conjure up a meal they couldn't serve.

Heavy, hand-pulled carts were used to haul goods to and from market stalls; bicycles and cars manoeuvred around them.

Poda-podas loaded passengers in front of the Rio. Some drivers took off at reckless speeds. I got better at keeping my wits about me when walking on streets with open gutters. I followed the zig-zagged lead of other pedestrians, dodging vehicles and stray dogs. The only semblance of a traffic jam in Bo was drivers waiting in line for fuel to arrive from Freetown.

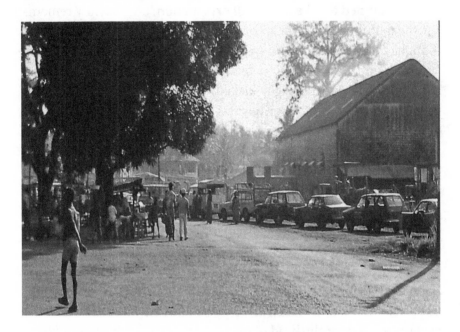

Vehicles lined up for petrol in Bo during one of the many periods of fuel shortages.

An Unexpected Proposal

I occasionally passed through Kenema, the provincial capital for the Eastern Province, en route to Segbwema Hospital, where Serabu's twinned SECHN training operated. Kenema was a transport hub where I had to transfer to a vehicle heading north. I received an astonishing proposition on one of those trips.

I was sitting on a low wooden bench in the back of a *poda-poda* in Kenema's lorry park, waiting for the driver to load other passengers. Mulling over my upcoming work in Segbwema, I was oblivious to activities around me. I didn't see the two men approaching until they appeared at the back of the truck. The older Pa, with a grin that revealed his missing teeth, was dressed in the regalia of a Paramount Chief. He was accompanied by a fit-looking, younger man, who I presumed was his appointed Speaker. Following Mende greetings and confirmation of their status, the Chief made a request. I could not understand his Mende. His straight-faced Speaker translated. I was too stunned to take in the full explanation, but I vividly remember the main message. The Chief had seen me across the lorry park, thought I was beautiful, and wanted to marry me.

Jolted out of my quiet reflections, I tried to hide my shock. A cultural-sensitivity trigger kicked in. I needed to treat the proposed betrothal with the seriousness the Chief must have thought it deserved. How to manage this social predicament? Without sensing my bewilderment, the Speaker continued, explaining emphatically that the Chief was offering a substantial bride-price including goats and cows. *My God,* I thought, *he's dead serious.*

I'm not sure from where my rebuttal idea came. It was driven by images of my father that flashed before me. This engagement, into what was undoubtedly a polygamous family, was not what my dad had in mind for his eldest daughter. With the Speaker acting as our interlocutor, I thanked the Chief for his generous offer and informed him that my father lived in Canada. As was customary, the bride-price was for the head of my household. The Chief would have to pay for the goats and cows to be flown air freight to Vancouver. The marriage deal was abruptly off. The Chief sauntered away a bit too nonplussed.

Fast-forward years later to when I was enjoying a family celebration the night before my wedding. That's when my fiancé gifted my father two plastic farm sets of animals. My fiancé had upped the bride-price offered by the Chief, albeit with plastic rather than live goods. Dad, who knew nothing of my marriage proposal in the lorry park, determined that my fiancé had gone bonkers.

Transportation Risks Brought into Focus

That most of the vehicles I rode in got to their destinations was remarkable. Breakdowns were common; poor vehicle maintenance issues were part of the problem. Bald tires, worn-out brakes, failing transmissions, and filthy exhaust fumes were the norm. Drivers did not carry spare tires; a flat meant a roadside wait. Sometimes we were rescued by a passing vehicle.

Bumpe Chiefdom had no garages, no tow trucks, and no fully-fledged mechanics. Bo was the closest location for any substantial vehicle repair work. I was mystified as to how drivers got broken-down vehicles with mechanical failures to the city.

Bad roads and too much daredevil driving contributed to road accidents. Although we had been warned of this during CUSO orientation sessions, and saw twisted steel carnage of accidents on roadsides, volunteers at Serabu Hospital rarely talked of this risk. I dared not imagine such a worst-case scenario. Given my duties, I was a passenger or a driver in a vehicle almost every day I spent in the villages. Travel risks were part of my community health job.

Eighteen months into my stay, the unthinkable happened. Carl, a vibrant and well-liked, mid-20s Peace Corps volunteer, was riding his standard-issue motorbike en route to Serabu when he lost control and hit a lorry head-on. He died instantly; news of his death left the volunteers visibly shaken. That he had even been issued a motorbike by Peace Corps authorities really rankled. Carl steered the motorbike with his one good arm. His other arm was paralyzed and hung in a sling; his significant disability the result of a motorcycle accident he had survived in the United States. My colleagues and I had worried that he'd lose control of his bike on the washboard-like laterite roads.

News of Carl's deplorable accident made the entire public health team acutely aware of our day-to-day travel risks. On the anniversary of his death, Carl's still distraught parents travelled to Kpetema, the village in Bumpe Chiefdom where he had been posted. His parents had paid for a well to be dug in his remembrance. I was told that the villagers honoured him during the memorial, with the respect they showed for Mende dignitaries.

A few months after Carl's tragic passing, I narrowly escaped a bad motor vehicle accident. Another one of my nine lives was used up. I remember the sequence of events like it happened yesterday. I was travelling back to Serabu from Freetown with Frank, a Dutch volunteer who was the foreman for hospital maintenance work. We had taken one *poda-poda* to Bo, where we had to transfer to another vehicle to get home. After getting into the back of the connecting *poda-poda*, I complained that I was parched. We climbed out to buy soft drinks in the Rio Restaurant. We were annoyed that "our" *poda-poda* driver took off without us.

Frank and I nabbed another vehicle after a short wait. As we neared the junction on Bo's outskirts, where the road to Serabu branched off, we saw a crowd gathering and ominous black smoke. Our driver slowed and then stopped. We gawked and shrieked at the ghastly site before us. The same *poda-poda* that Frank and I had originally boarded outside the Rio had slammed into a tanker truck. Both vehicles were over-turned; the tanker smouldered. We piled out and joined other hushed onlookers. Several dead bodies were strewn on the ground. A few bystanders carried badly injured passengers to safety.

Although memory tells me that an ambulance arrived, I may have conjured up that image from a sense of surviving-nurse guilt. The scene was gruesome. Neither Frank nor I stepped in to assist. I did not offer any trauma care. Instead, we stood well back on the sidelines, shaking shoulder to shoulder, and muttering exclamations of disbelief and shock. We furtively asked each other whether or not to intervene. Our driver was agitated and anxious to leave the scene. After a short time that seemed to last forever, he urgently waved us back into his *poda-poda*. We drove away.

For the rest of the trip to Serabu, I was silent and sullen. My mind was numb. When we arrived back, I went straight to the convent and spewed out my bottled-up anguish to Sister Hilary, describing the horrific scene and how it had immobilized me. She was thankful that Frank and I were safe and sympathetic to how I had reacted at the crash site.

I scrolled through the mental images and the eerie feeling of that accident scene hundreds of times. Frank and I had been onlookers, fearful for our own lives should the tanker explode, and stunned with the knowledge that we had narrowly escaped being among the ill-fated passengers.

Something inside me changed. Our near-miss locked an element of fatalism into my travelling mindset. *Eh deh to God.* It hadn't been my time to die. I had no other reasonable explanation.

Chapter 9
Play, Learning, and Celebrations

I formed early but distorted impressions of children's play. It appeared more happenstance than deliberate. Mothers involved little ones in their day-to-day chores and created play out of work. I thought play-forms lacked diversity.

My observations were blinkered by the lack of toys: no picture books; no blocks; no Lego; no Fisher-Price gear; no wind-up toys; no board games; no puzzles; no Play-Doh, crayons, or colouring books; no stuffed animals or Barbie dolls; and no ride-em toys or tricycles. I had considered age-appropriate toys to be essential for play and education.

Play Forms

Infants and toddlers moved as one with their mothers, whether swaddled on their backs, hoisted on their hips, sitting on their laps, or walking by their sides. Toddlers and young children were never out of sight. Siblings and other women watched, comforted, amused, and encouraged youngsters. Young school-age children were put on care-giving duty; their dolls were live babies. Mothers strapped infants and toddlers onto the backs of older brothers or sisters with *lappas*. Training in child care was part of play.

Play never involved a high-tech interface. There was no putting a little one in front of a television, radio, record player, or tape recorder to let a gadget amuse or distract. Electronic toys had entertained my younger siblings when they were preschoolers. My brother could hardly contain his laughter when he watched Winnie the Pooh movies, and my younger sister knew all the *Sesame Street* puppets. In the villages, the only electronic gadgets were battery-operated, short-wave radios. These were adult devices, not instruments of play.

I saw homemade toys: sticks to propel old bike tire rims, wire bent in the shape of a lorry, sling shots used for target games, and slit drums made of bamboo cane. They reminded me of the playthings Dad had made for my sister and me: a swing set with the supporting structure fashioned from tree trunks, a wheelbarrow that was a recycled masterpiece. Dad pushed us around as we rode on top of crisp autumn leaves. I, too, had enjoyed the play value of recycled toys in my childhood.

Play among pre-teens looked gendered. I saw boys, not girls, using homemade toys. I wondered if school-age girls were too busy with women's work for light-hearted playtime. Gendered roles were reinforced at a young age.

I reflected on my childhood. The assignment of household chores had been determined by age not gender. I could never understand the depths of gendered roles in Mende society. Offering my commentary on gendered activities seemed out of place. Who was I to critique or opine on what children played with, who got to play, and how household chores were divided between girls and boys?

Pets

Families did not have pets. However, animals were in every village: always chickens and goats, often dogs and cats. They wandered freely, scavenging food. Dogs generally looked scrawny and uncared for. It was hard to accept the survival-of-the-fittest attitude towards animals.

Young children were kinder than adults with domestic animals; soothing them with touch and words. They grasped the fundamentals of animal care through playful connections. Curiosity fuelled children's interests in other creatures. They saw plenty of them in villages, on farms, and in streams and swamps. Learning how to live alongside critters and figuring out which were safe and which were not was a vital skill. Sometimes I was the intended beneficiary of youngsters' animal capture escapades. Pre-teens showed up at my house one day with a live turtle, enthusiastically selling it for *best price*. I declined.

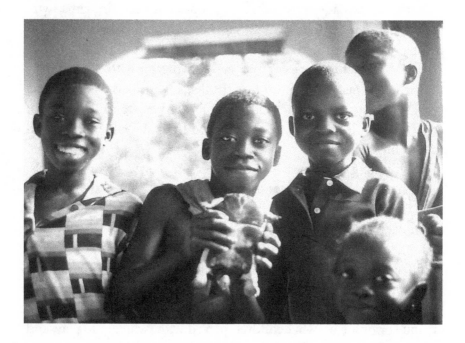

Children offering to sell me a turtle on the veranda of my village home in Serabu.

School

Most youngsters walked long distances to primary school. Families had scarcely enough money for school fees and uniforms; paying a *poda-poda* driver to transport their *piken* to or from school was unthinkable. I wondered if young pupils dawdled en route.

I was shocked to see how ultra-bare-boned primary schools were. They contained simple furnishings: worn benches for writing and sitting, and chalkboards made of planed wood that had been painted black. The simplest of teaching aids—like letters of the alphabet or word cards on walls—were missing. Parent-teacher nights weren't a thing.

Rote learning was the modus operandi. When a primary school was in session, I'd hear the sing-song-like repetition of arithmetic tables, the alphabet, or word passages. Initially, I assumed rote-teaching left students bored and disinterested. However, even children in the earliest grades understood that attending school was a special privilege. Youngsters approached their lessons with gusto.

Primary teachers had no educational resources to prompt learning through play. Teachers did their best, building on the strong and vibrant oral tradition of Mende society. I reminded myself that all of Serabu's nursing students had succeeded with the same type of formative teaching.

School teachers used the pedagogical methods they had experienced as pupils. Multi-grade classes looked full, even though only a small fraction of village children went to school. The primary school teachers I met were committed to their role and determined to improve literacy levels. They envisioned more children advancing to secondary school with better employment opportunities that could release families from poverty. I admired teachers' enthusiasm and perseverance. They had a tough job.

Games

Clapping, tag, and other group games were common. I relived a bit of my own youth when I saw kids energetically play games during school recesses and in their villages. Soccer matches were held in a large field by the main road in Serabu. Most children played in bare feet, and the soccer ball was fashioned out of tied rags. Onlookers cheered for their team.

Teachers organized athletic days. I was impressed by the high jumpers, especially those who confidently launched themselves over the bamboo bar in bare feet. As a child, my performance in this sport had been dismal and that was without the challenge of a shoeless running start.

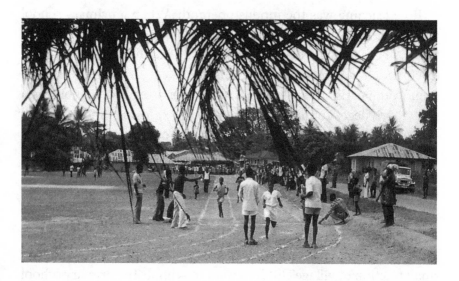

Athletics' day, Serabu village.

Informal games accompanied women's chores. Children splashed and cavorted in streams and rivers while their mothers laundered clothes, keeping little ones within visual range. The women assembled in groups, *lappas* hoisted thigh-high in the shallows. They rubbed clothes and bedding with soap and settled into the rhythm of beating and kneading items on rocks for a thorough cleansing. Laundry was draped over trees and bushes to dry.

Nearby, older kids showed younger ones how to paddle. No one taught life-saving skills. Watching their water play made me feel like jumping in, but that play domain was for children. Adults' connections with water were for the necessities of life: bathing, laundering, drinking-water retrieval, fishing, and transportation. I wondered if women secretly longed for frivolous splash time.

Male adolescents watched and sometimes took part in betting games organized by men; their games' tables consisted of bald tires covered with woven mats on which small wooden tops were spun. Players and observers gathered round, watching intensely. I never saw girls or women join betting games. I speculated that they disapproved of gambling sidelines and the palm wine that was passed around, which upped the bets wagered.

Teens and young adults played Mancala on a carved wooden board with seeds or stones. This was the only pseudo-board game I recognized. In my youth, learning how to play Monopoly, Clue, and Risk had been a rite-of-passage. In the villages, strategy was taught to youth in ways I didn't see.

Chores

Life skills were learned through everyday living. It did not surprise me that preschoolers eagerly helped with chores. Their enthusiasm out-matched their physical strength and coordination. Young children were play-acting; learning how to contribute to family life.

My curiosity was piqued by older children. I never heard them argue with parents about doing chores. School-aged children carried water, fetched firewood, sold fruit, swept dirt floors, picked crops, and helped thresh and winnow rice and sorghum grains. Led by women, pre-teens were shown how to corral small fish into nets. Everyone mastered bird-scaring techniques used during harvest time.

Women were trailed by school-age children as they balanced scrappy buckets and jerry cans on their heads, carrying water for drinking and cooking. Head ties, shaped like protective donuts, rested on their plaited hair. Taut neck cords steadied their full loads; no splashes, no wastage. Children carried partially filled buckets. They were learning by doing.

I don't know at what age these activities morphed from play to work. Children's attitudes towards their chores did not demarcate this change. They didn't do chores to earn rewards or pocket money. Rather, chores were about getting by, day-to-day. Subsistence living required all hands on deck.

Hair Braiding

I was fascinated by the intricate hair braiding of girls and women. A household's well-worn wooden comb was used to divide the hair, creating a canvass for the symmetrical, geometric, and swirling patterns of braids. This universal grooming practice started when females were babies. As they grew older, girls graduated from simple to complicated hair designs.

Sitting on a stool or on the ground, the child or adult whose hair was being braided rested her head on the lap or knee of the braider. The braider's fingers moved deftly, like expert knitters without the needles. The duo slipped into a peaceful interlude of comradery and connectedness. Even preschoolers were still and quiet as their hair was sculpted; so different from the tussles I had with my young sister when I brushed her long hair. Among the Mende, braiding provided women with protected time; brief and welcome respites from their heavy work.[12]

Older women had their hair braided for special ceremonies. For adolescents and young women such as my students, everyday braids were an elaborate, individualized statement of beauty. In some girls' secondary boarding schools, principals limited the amount of time for hair-braiding when it depleted attention to homework. It seemed a shame that female nursing students had to partially cover their ornate hair designs with a cap.

Hair braiding was as much an art form on carved *sowos* (*Bundu* masks) as on the heads of young girls and women. These helmet-shaped, blackened masks featured rows and rows of intricate braids painstakingly carved into the wood. Each completed mask was a cultural icon, worn by a *Sowei* during Secret Society ceremonies that only *Bundu* members could attend.[13] Occasionally, a *sowo* was worn in public. Word would quickly spread that the *Bundu* devil was going to be *pulled*. For public dancing, a *Sowei* wore the sacred *sowo* and a costume made of black raffia and cloth that completely covered her body. A small entourage guided the *Bundu* devil as she danced on village paths.

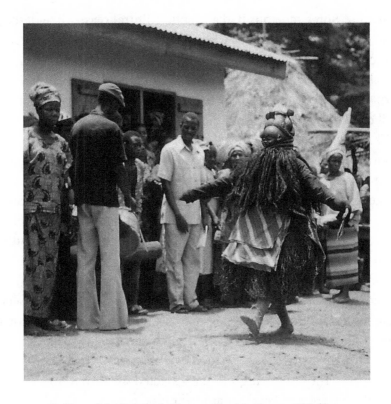

Pulling of the Bundu devil at a village in Bumpe Chiefdom.

For me, these celebratory gatherings were mysterious and haunting. They were overt reminders that I was an outsider to the Mende culture. I felt privileged to have seen *sowo* icons up close and in context.

Stories, Celebrations, Music, and Dance

Values were taught through examples and stories. Mende fables were rich with the imagery of creatures like spiders, turtles, and monkeys that lived in fantastical places. My students knew these tales by heart, even though they had never seen written or illustrated versions of them. Local fables had stirred their imaginations, while offering lessons about the origins of humankind, the mysteries of life, and the wisdom of elders. Like Aesop's fables, Mende fables conveyed moral tensions: generosity versus greed, and honest versus corrupt behaviour. Some tensions had a Mende cultural twist—like descriptions of mean protagonists whose actions served personal rather than collective interests.

Celebrations were playful times. Young and old partook; farm-work duties were put aside. I soaked up the delicious displays of devil costumes and swayed to the rhythms of song and dance.

Children and adults dressed up as village devils. Costume-wise, this was the closest we got to Halloween. Youngsters made costumes using cloth remnants discarded by tailors or used clothing sold in markets. Thick, draped layers of raffia were part of the attire. Shells sewn or tied onto the outfits provided a distinctive rattle as devils moved and danced. Simple cloth head-coverings or masks made of wood completed the getup.

Some costumes mimicked the formal tradition of devil masquerades; important initiation rituals of the *Bundu* and *Poro* Secret Societies.[14] Heavy wooden *jilo* masks amused. They were torso- rather than head-size and gave the adult wearer a clown-like appearance, with their huge, oval-shaped eye holes and thick lips painted with ochre. Those wearing *jilo* masks acted as mimes and comics, generating ripples of laughter among onlookers.

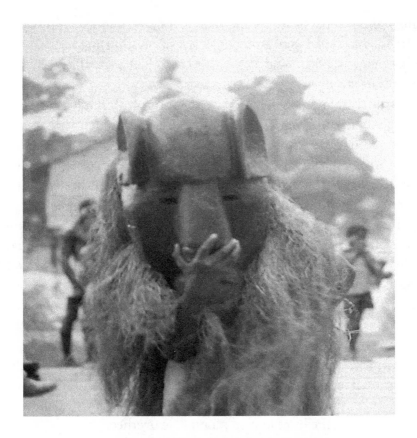

Heavy, wooden jilo mask worn by a young man.

Children danced alongside adults dressed as devils, sometimes as their accomplices. Simple props were used for a bit of trickery. Two kids dressed in costume came into the common room of our home on Christmas day. One play-acted as a deer, the other as a hunter. The hunter pretended to shoot the deer. We were not sure how to move the performers along and, more specifically, out of our house. It dawned on us that a small *dash* (bribe) was the revival trick. Off they went, mission accomplished.

Teens added hilarity to devil dancing, parading among crowds on tall wooden stilts. Little ones hugged their mother's legs, frightened by the tall creatures, but giggling nonetheless.

The music and singing made me tingle with delight. Women sang in harmony as they pounded food in mortars, worked in the fields, and announced a birth. Drums, wooden flutes, and *segburas* (gourd rattles also called *shake-shakes*) were played during celebrations. Like me, children found it hard to keep their feet still when they heard the steady beat of local rhythms.

Formal training in dance was part of the girl's *Bundu* initiation. For celebrations, groups of adolescent girls and women were unified in dance and dress; their *oshobi* (matching) outfits made with bold West African prints. I found their upper-body swings, gyrating hip motions, and leg-stepping rhythms fast-paced and evocative. Their dance moves were a Mende art form I was unable to mimic.

I was enthralled by the rich harmonies of Mende songs. A lead sang the chants. An entourage responded by answering in refrain or with a chorus. Singing continued for long stretches of time, generating a comforting aura. Singers and onlookers shuffled along, absorbing the musical beat, forming a gently propelled conga dance line. When asked to join, I was abundantly conscious of my awkward *pomwei* moves.

A musical interlude of another kind took place on clear nights when a full moon cast its light. Children were allowed to stay up well past their customary bedtime. A kinetic percussion instrumental would start as the luminescent moon rose overhead. Youngsters celebrated enthusiastically, banging metal objects under the communal glow. Despite being distant from my family, I mused that we were all part of humankind, generating cosmic connections in the same grand universe.

Christmas Magic

Christmas was a difficult time to be so far from home. Serabu's expatriate community sensed the tug of family and kin. The only visible symbol of Christmas was the nativity scene in the church.

Mass was celebrated on Christmas Eve. A lump lodged in my throat when the congregation turned to watch the chorus of women make their way up the aisle as they sang the traditional birth song in multi-part harmonies, carrying a small rag doll, baby *Jesuis*, up to the nativity.

Christmas day began with a visit to the children's ward, where the Sisters and volunteers gave out cubes of sugar, cans of sweetened milk, and *groundnuts*. Although patients and their families came from predominantly or exclusively Muslim or animist villages and knew little of Christmas, their eyes sparkled as presents were shared.

Serabu was spruced up for Christmas Day. Yards were swept with extra care. Many dressed in their finest; that is, the one outfit they owned that was not used for farming work. Devils danced on the street.

Some years we had unexpected arrivals. Not all were welcome, as Christmas week was a period when the Sisters and volunteers sought a bit of downtime. One Christmas Eve, two unannounced visitors (a British journalist and a medical doctor from Argentina) arrived at 10 PM asking to be shown around the hospital. I was underwhelmed by their audacity.

Another year, Connie and I planned Christmas dinner for an invited crowd of 24 volunteers. We ordered pseudo-turkeys (very small chickens) from the farm in Walihun and prepared three ovens: iron cooking pots perched over three-stone fires. We made pumpkin pies for dessert, with enough slices to satisfy our hungry guests.

New Year's Eve was celebrated with a large bonfire, singing, and storytelling beside the convent. Serabu's international volunteers and Sisters welcomed in the New Year with a toast to a better future for the people of Sierra Leone.

PART 3
PRIMARY HEALTH CARE

"Who could be so lucky? Who comes to a lake for water and sees the reflection of moon?" (Rumi)

CHAPTER 10
CLASSROOM AND FIELDWORK

The CUSO position I had applied for was that of public health tutor. I assumed my teaching would be in the classroom rather than in the field. My job was not quite as advertised. The first cohort of SECHN students had started their final phase of community health training before my arrival. Nancy Reimer had taken on the classroom instruction. My main responsibilities had shifted to supervising students' fieldwork. My fragile confidence bubble burst.

This was the first of several job changes, prompted by a revolving door of international volunteers. Nancy developed pregnancy complications. She and her husband had to leave Serabu a few months after I arrived. I took on her teaching, with a day's notice. Dale arrived a few months after Nancy's departure. She picked up fieldwork responsibilities. After a dozen weeks on the job, Dale was medevacked. A bout of dysentery had triggered Dale's pre-existing health condition. Once again, I shifted gears. Anne, a third Peace Corps nurse arrived months later. She was assigned to classroom teaching. After a year in Serabu, she had to return home for treatment of a recurring medical condition. Connie, a CUSO, volunteer arrived towards the end of my second year. She took on fieldwork supervision and stayed for three years. During Connie's tenure, Winkie, a third CUSO nurse became critically ill. Another medevac. Another blow to the stability of expatriates for Serabu's public health team.

Since students were either in the classroom or in the field, and only one cohort of students completed the community health segment of their training at any one time, double-duty job expectations were manageable in the short-term. Nevertheless, staff changes were unsettling. The fragility of our international community health workforce was ever-present. Recruiting volunteers was a lengthy, drawn-out process.

Our public health team was poking its fingers into the holes of a leaking human resource dike. For me, navigating these workforce limitations built a stronger sense of comradery with my Sierra Leonean colleagues. I tried to focus my attention on the long-term aspiration of robust Sierra Leonean public health nursing capacity.

Serabu's primary health care program was growing rapidly. Village health needs outstripped our capacity. The workload was heavy. What had been a one-man Sierra Leonean public health team when I first arrived, expanded with several new hires, including Simeon Tucker, an experienced enrolled nurse, and then John and Thomas who were early graduates of Serabu's SECHN training. Marcella Reffell, a village maternity assistant with plenty of clinical know-how also joined. She supported Sister Denise Dorr with TBA training and mobile prenatal clinics.

Sierra Leonean staff led primary health care fieldwork and took on the role of preceptors for students. They were the dependable employees of Serabu Hospital. Unlike the international volunteers, they were engaged for the long-haul. No end-of-placement contract date hovered over them.

Sister Hilary provided steady leadership as we weathered personnel changes. But she too, had to work around gaps in physician coverage. When Sister Sheila Kelly, the hospital's lead surgeon, left for Ireland to complete her surgical residency, Sister Hilary was thrown back into the operating room. David, the newly-arrived CUSO physician, had Mama Hilary alongside as he mastered new surgical skills and assumed administrative roles.

I figured out ways to get her guidance, which I badly needed. On days when I was in the office, Sister Hilary often dropped by after completing her last surgical case and before heading up to the convent for lunch. I had my pedantic questions ready. She usually began by recounting a challenging or satisfying surgical case. I especially recall her accounts of repair surgery for women who suffered from a condition I'd never seen in Canada. Vesico-vaginal fistulas are a nasty complication of a lengthy period of obstructed labour. A small passage opens up between the bladder or rectum and vagina, leaking urine or feces. Surgical repairs of fistulas are intricate and risky. Successful repairs could alter the life courses of women who had been shunned in their communities due to incontinence. Sister Hilary's descriptions of these surgical cases left me in awe. Her extraordinary talents ran deep and wide, bridging leading-edge surgical techniques and vanguard strategies for prevention.

I needed Sister Hilary's creative and analytical mind for bigger issues and ideas concerning Serabu's burgeoning primary health care program. I arranged to travel with her when she went to Bo on business. Mama Hilary was always offered a soft-cushioned seat in the cab, where I'd sit beside her, using every minute of the ride to turn her undivided attention to program challenges. Our *poda-poda* journeys provided odd conversational conditions. The Krio banter between the driver and his apprentice, who book-ended us on the bench seat, didn't get in the way of our essential dialogue. Each trip with Sister Hilary left me reinfused with her resolute determination to deliver primary health care to the communities of Bumpe Chiefdom.

Classroom Teaching

SECHN training was 30 months long. Male and female students completed the first 17 months together during which they focused on general nursing, including medical, surgical, and pediatric care for inpatients. Female students then completed an eight-month midwifery component in Segbwema, while male students continued in the generic segment with some public health learning, such as how to run outpatient clinics. In the last five months, all students came back together to study community health in Serabu.

We immersed students in disease prevention and health promotion theory and practice. Students were enthusiastic. Their registration exams and certification were within reach; they were excited to use and expand upon their nursing skills outside the confines of the hospital. They readily took to the work.

A strong community health training component marked a big leap forward to address the health realities of rural Sierra Leone. Student nurses from Freetown were required to complete a short clinical placement with Serabu's primary health care initiative.

I began classroom instruction with a pittance of local clinical experience. I fretted about the relevance of my Canadian community health examples. I was alert to cues indicating my Western-oriented approaches were faulty or inappropriate. The content of my instruction rested too heavily on the small shelf of reference books in my office. Like my students, I felt the climb of a learning trajectory when I prepared lessons on assessing community needs, engaging village leaders, and working with health committees.

While students were new to the theory of public health, most had grown up in villages. All had a solid grounding in clinical practice, albeit in hospital settings. Through trial and error, I learned how to draw on the students' experiential foundations as we considered community health challenges and debated fundamental principles of public health. I began to see my primary teaching role as that of a facilitator. I could help students develop a lens to re-examine their clinical practice and revisit their understanding of poverty, illiteracy, power dynamics, and community engagement. Interactive strategies like role-plays gave students an opportunity to try out new skills and allowed me to delve into nuances of cultural communication. I was a learner in the process.

Missed Opportunities

The reality of a thin and transient workforce capacity squelched discussions about having Sierra Leonean counterparts either for me or the other public health tutors. Sierra Leonean community health nurses were maxed out with work responsibilities in the villages. While any one of them could have filled in for international tutors in the classroom, we could not replace them in the villages. We lacked the requisite Mende language skills and cultural know-how.

I look back at missed opportunities with chagrin. I rarely invited Sierra Leonean public health staff to teach in the classroom. I could have passed on techniques for planning lessons and curricula, or evaluating students' knowledge and skills. My colleagues would have enriched classroom learning.

When I had to shift job responsibilities, I operated in crisis mode. This narrowed my thinking. I did not always walk the talk of sustainable development.

Best Laid Plans

I was constantly planning public health practice opportunities for students. Village circumstances could change abruptly, necessitating on-the-spot adjustments. Over a few days, when I and other senior public health staff were away from Serabu, a series of events played havoc with carefully laid plans.

Journal Entry

Circa January, 1981

Near-chaos reigned while we were gone.

The TBAs in Magema are away for a burial ceremony, so the Chief refuses to allow the two female nursing students to stay in the village overnight.

In Bongor, the *Poro* Society celebrations are on—the *Poro* devil is out. Anybody who is not a member must stay indoors. No health committee meetings can be held, no visits can be made.

Two female nursing students are needed for roles in the health education drama in Bongor. They refuse to go because of *Poro* celebrations.

The driver takes the students who are supposed to be going to Makoba and Mokpendeh as far as Bongor but then refuses to take them further because of the *Poro* celebrations.

Fifteen nursing students arrive from Freetown with no advance notice. Sister Hilary sends them off to Bongor, bringing the total number of students in that village up to 30.

Thomas, [our newly hired public health staff member], asks what I would have done had I been there. I tell him: "Send them walking to surrounding villages with a report to write." We enjoy a good laugh.

Any student learning that had taken place in our absence had little to do with our planning efforts. The scenarios that unfolded were another reminder that accommodating the unexpected was a critical public health competency.

Peripheral Health Units

While the challenges we experienced in the classroom and field could be vexing, our public health team had the support of a well-run hospital that was adequately staffed, with a reasonably consistent supply of drugs and equipment. Serabu Hospital worked within and alongside a government system of peripheral health units that were scattered across Bumpe Chiefdom. We frequently interacted with peripheral health unit government employees. They had a different work reality.

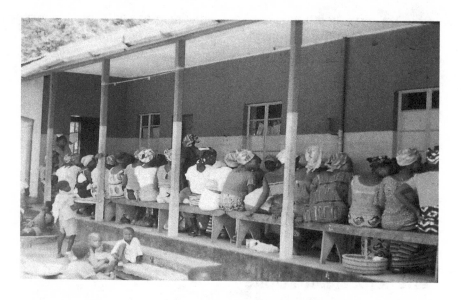

Women waiting to be seen by the dispenser and MCH aide in an antenatal and under-five clinic held in a government health centre.

No replacement staff were readily available for deployment if a health worker vacated their post or fell sick. Rare supervisory visits by more qualified provincial health workers were often for discipline rather than support. Continuing education opportunities were few and far between.

Peripheral health unit staff were expected to refer difficult cases to the hospital. They had no way to call for a consult when a medical emergency occurred. They would try to summon local transport for patients needing urgent attention.

Health and treatment centre staff worked within the confines of a frugal infrastructure and limited equipment and supplies. There was little government funding for either maintaining buildings or constructing add-ons like latrines or wells. Some health and treatment centres were in a bad state of repair. One centre had been overtaken by bats. Its ceiling tiles were rotted and putrid with bat excrement. Staff had moved their clinic services to the dispenser's home. I found their work environments dark, dank, depressing, and demotivating. Yet, they forged on.

Dispensers and EDCU assistants were responsible for collecting whatever drugs, supplies, and replacement equipment they needed from the Ministry's central stores in Freetown. Given the distance from Bumpe Chiefdom to the capital, these return trips took at least two work-days each month. Workers made the tiring journey on *poda-podas*. Their trips were exceedingly frustrating when they came back empty-handed or short of basic supplies, like thermometers or clinic registers, and essential drugs like chloroquine, iron tablets, ergometrine, and antibiotics. Central supply stock-outs were common. Word quickly got out when peripheral health unit staff had no drugs to treat common conditions. Clinic attendance dropped; trust eroded. Rebounding was tough going.

A drop in clinic revenue made government staff's perilous salary situation worse. Collecting monthly paycheques involved a trip to the payroll office in the provincial capital; though there was no certainty salaries would be paid on time. Their erratic and low-wage income forced them into sidelines of work like farming, so they could feed their own families. Most staff were committed to their health work and engaged in local community life. However, work demands took an emotional toll, reduced morale, and sometimes fractured relationships among peripheral health unit staff and with villagers.

For MCH aides and village maternity assistants deployed to villages that were designated as health posts, conditions were even more basic. The government did not build clinic facilities in these communities. Rather, local village authorities were expected to provide health workers with a clinic room and lodging. Clinic rooms were small and austere, and usually under the same roof as the health worker's private and meagre living quarters.

Furnishings were minimalist. A small wooden cot was used for antenatal examinations and deliveries. Fully equipped meant having a blood-pressure cuff, stethoscope, rubber ground sheet, wooden fetoscope, infant weigh scale, thermometer, bucket, a pair of forceps and scissors, and a small kettle to sterilize equipment on a three-stone fire. MCH aides had a few drugs like chloroquine, aspirin, folic acid, and ferrous sulfate to treat common conditions.

Maternity staff showed pride of ownership. They whitewashed undulating mud walls to deter insects, swept the cement or earthen floors, and hung cloths on window frames for a bit of privacy. Sparse supplies were tidily arranged on rustic tables. On clinic days, MCH aides proudly wore their dusty-pink uniforms, white bib-aprons, and small nursing caps.

MCH aides and village maternity assistants received a stipend rather than a salary from government. Payment for the deliveries they attended, whether in cash or in kind, came from the families of patients. That was their main source of income. They received scant supervision but often joined Serabu Hospital staff when mobile clinics were held in their villages.

Peripheral health unit staff did not have the buffering support of others or the day-to-day comradery of more qualified health workers that Serabu Hospital staff enjoyed. All eyes and expectations of the villagers they served were on them 24/7. When obstetrical emergencies occurred, MCH aides and village maternity assistants must have sensed utter isolation and frantic distress. Their work circumstances set them up for colossal patient care failures.

CHAPTER 11
REVAMPING
COMMUNITY ASSESSMENTS

When Sister Hilary initiated the primary health care pilot in three small villages, physical assessments of all community residents were undertaken and repeated annually for several years. Stage II program expansion into section villages required a do-over of the assessment approach to lessen resource requirements.

Sister Hilary and I wanted to capture indicators of health status while engaging villagers in dialogue about their community's health-related needs. Sharing assessment results was intended to prompt villagers and their leaders to think anew about old problems, while surfacing health priorities. One main principle guided us: Knowledge is power, the power for change.

David Werner's text, *Where There is No Doctor*, was my go-to resource. The pages detailing community assessments started to look dog-eared. Dr. Werner outlined questions to tap perceived strengths and needs, community history, and leadership.

Our assessment would be experience-informed rather than record-rich since written records were sparse. No written history of local communities and no village-specific data on immunizations, antenatal visits, births, deaths, water and sanitation infrastructure, or harvest yields were available. No clinical summaries were kept by traditional healers or birth attendants. Serabu Hospital's annual reports provided a snapshot of common diagnoses but only among those seeking treatment either as inpatients or outpatients.

The new assessment approach was led by Serabu's public health staff. Students assisted. Elders shared the oral history of their village.

TBAs recounted their midwifery practice. Chiefs and other village leaders were asked about farming; getting produce to market; common health woes; and the availability of latrines, safe drinking water sources, schools, and literacy classes. We inquired about problems and solutions.

With the assistance of TBAs, Serabu's public health team completed a census and queried all households about illnesses, births, and deaths. Mothers and pregnant women were asked about clinic attendance. Family-retained immunization cards were reviewed. Visual checks were made for Bacille Calmette-Guérin (BCG) vaccination scars. Nurses measured the circumference of children's upper arms using thin strips of old X-ray film, marked off to indicate red, yellow, and green zones; identifying those who were severely or marginally malnourished.

Accurate dates are needed to estimate birth, mortality, and morbidity rates in the past year, and whether to categorize the death of a child as a neonatal (within first 28 days of life), infant (within first year of life), or under-five death. This was not straight-forward. I had taken the use of a Gregorian calendar for granted. But a calendar is useless when you can't read. I had not considered how frequently clinical questions were linked to specific times and dates.

I had expected people to know their date of birth. While births were cause for celebration, birthdays were not. Few births were registered. Families rarely had a confirmatory birth record. When infants were immunized, the birthdate was estimated using a local calendar.

Villagers tracked years with major happenings: the great earthquake, coronations or deaths of Paramount Chiefs, the country's independence. An annual calendar consisted of approximate dates for seasonal rains and *dries*; slashing and burning the bush, harvesting rice; religious and Secret Society ceremonies; primary school terms; and annual hut tax collection. An infant's naming ceremony took place around the seventh day of life. Forty-day mourning periods followed deaths. These occurrences provided the chronological structure for local calendars, guiding questions about the timing of illnesses, births, and deaths.

Household interviews could be intense. We were delving into the highs and lows of community life. Some stories were heart-warming: A premature infant nursed back to health. Families with school-age children, who had all survived their early years. A young woman who had birthed healthy twins. Kids fully immunized for their age. A polygamous household head adamant that his pregnant wives regularly attend clinic.

Too often, we had to probe for heart-wrenching details of untimely deaths, gathering information about causes, ages, and dates. Mothers saddened as they remembered little ones lost. Granny midwives trembled as they gave harrowing details of mothers who had died in childbirth.

We maintained that communities were owners of the information collected. I tabulated responses and summarized data in a short community report with simple tables and graphs. Death rates in many villages left me incredulous. One third of all newborns died before they reached 12 months of age; 40% of all children died before they reached the age of five. I would check and double-check the incomprehensible numbers.

When analysis was complete, nurses who had collected data headed back to the village to share results. A short written report was given to the Chief. Data-sharing events were well-attended; every household had participated. Illiteracy didn't hold them back. The Village Chief usually began by asking us to confirm the number of men and women who lived in the village, thereby initiating the two-sided reveal.

Villagers got new information about their community. Our public health team gained insights from villagers' intimate knowledge of their local situation. Assessment results provided an entry-point to explore how villagers, public health staff, and students could work together on health improvements and the possibility of setting up a village health committee.

Power Struggles

The health data we gathered were robust. However, I wasn't sure we were tapping into less tangible aspects of village life such as leadership. The lineage of Village and Paramount Chiefs was a backbone for governance, but I found its subtleties difficult to grasp. I knew that leaders could make or break our primary health care efforts.

The approach we had adopted to assess leadership was right out of David Werner's textbook. It was simple; possibly simplistic. We asked the Village Chief to direct us to the household head who should relay the village's history. We had questions ready. What were the origins of the village? Who initially settled here? How did the village get its name? I wondered if these assessment questions would uncover lineage disputes or infighting.

A Chief's unusual response suggested our questions were on the right track. He directed us to speak with two household heads about the village origins; a clue that something was amiss. The two households provided contradictory village histories. We had surfaced a simmering, lineage disagreement.

This dispute was playing out around the new village well and partly explained the lack of a common public bucket to draw water. Instead, the village had two buckets, which were stored in different homes. Villagers showed their disposition towards one lineage or the other based on the household from which they borrowed a bucket. Uncertainty about leadership had generated mistrust in the community. Well-poisoning rumours were circulating.

Paul and Simeon filled in my cultural blanks. Threats of well-poisoning led families to avoid using a protected well, opting instead for traditional, albeit contaminated water sources. To the naked eye, well water appears to be a small, stagnant point source of water; perfect conditions for spiteful poisoning. Unresolved disputes heightened villagers' trepidation of willful malice like tampering with well water.

In contrast to wells, the visible flow of water in streams and rivers left families assured that should poisoning of a surface water source occur, the poison would soon dissipate. Furthermore, ancestors and spirits such as *tingoi* and *njaloi* were believed to provide protection for villages. These entities lived near traditional drinking water sources. They had to be treated properly through ceremonies and considerate day-to-day living. Drawing water from a well could be disrespectful. Malevolent poisoning of streams and rivers showed serious disregard for ancestors. Miffed ancestral spirits brought misfortune to a village. Nobody wanted to be responsible or blamed for an affront. Big stakes were involved.[15]

A development aid project to dig and encase a village well could go off the rails. Ancestors were custodians and purveyors of social harmony. I had included no questions about them in the community assessment.

The simple question we had asked the Chief about the custodian of the village's oral history had given us entrée into a dispute that threatened villagers' access to clean water. A small deviation from Chiefs' usual designation of a single oral historian in a village had provided an unexpected peek at a power struggle.

World Health Day

Although Chiefs were attentive when we shared assessment results during village feedback sessions, I thought it was unlikely the details stuck with them. My skepticism was blown to bits, suitably on a World Health Day. Local Chiefs had assembled to confer on Chiefdom matters. Serabu's public health team had set up a display about preventing childhood diseases in the *barrie*. Nurses were primed to facilitate an exchange among these leaders. Which villages were leading, and which were lagging, on immunizations and other health indicators, and why?

I was stunned when the Chiefs spontaneously began comparing data from their village assessments. With no prompting from our team, they debated how a few villages had managed to eradicate or reduce rates of *soin-soin* and *nyenye* (measles), and why some communities had higher rates of under-five deaths than others. We watched with pride as they challenged each other to get their women and children immunized and make other health improvements.

Unexpected and momentous occasions like these left me feeling certain that Serabu's primary health care efforts were making a difference. Tucked away, in the small village of Serabu, in a tiny corner of the world, I was part of a game-changing initiative.

CHAPTER 12
EXPECT THE UNEXPECTED

Fieldwork could go awry, undermined by unexpected events, unanticipated reactions, and village palavers or crises. Well-intentioned health messages could be distorted and planning diverted. Small successes kept us forging ahead. I was invigorated by surprising breakthroughs, bursts in momentum, and joined-up efforts.

Whether I had a bad or good field day, village work gave me pause. Taking stock, regrouping, readjusting, and re-planning were all part of moving on. Circumstances that left me frustrated were countered by situations that fuelled my optimism.

Village Protocols and Overnighters

Our public health team tried to cover all protocols to get permission for village work. We sent advance notification of planned visits. Women who came to clinic were asked to take messages back to their villages. We gave *poda-poda* drivers written notes to deliver. Runners were sent with letters to nearby communities. Unless someone in the village had English literacy skills, our messages went unread. Ultimately, the Chief or his/her delegate decided whether or not we could proceed. This decision was normally conveyed to us after we got to the community.

There were no hostels, bed and breakfast businesses, or guest rooms in the villages. Our overnight presence was an imposition. We displaced others from their beds and their mosquito nets, if they had them.

If I required overnight village lodging, a suitable room had to be found and other awkward matters dealt with like where a female *pomwei* could bathe, whether or not there was a usable latrine or an extra kerosene lamp available, and what unstated expectations I had. During my few overnight village stays, I was given rooms in the homes of primary school teachers and Village Chiefs.

When farming season was in full swing, we'd plan evening visits to share community assessment results, encourage village health committee members with their efforts, or conduct immunization clinics. After-dark visits were restricted to motorable villages; bush-walking at night was dangerous.

In predominantly Muslim villages, we'd sometimes arrive to the sound of prayer or see children gathered around a bonfire with an adult leading their recital of the Quran. On nights when rains were heavy, villages could appear deserted as families sought refuge around the glow of small open fires inside their homes.

Taninahun

Paul was sure all the right people had been informed as we set out to Taninahun. He had sent notes to the Section Chief, Town Chief, and dispenser via a *poda-poda* driver, indicating that Serabu's nurses and students were coming to discuss sanitation with their health committee.

We arrived at dusk. Paul and I asked students to wait in the *barrie*, while we set off to find the Section Chief. He was out of town. We were directed to the Town Chief. He was sick in bed and couldn't get up. We located the home of the health committee's Chairman; he was busy eating. His senior wife asked us to come back later. Next in the protocol hierarchy was the dispenser, who argued that he had not expected us during evening hours. After a terse exchange, we headed back to the Chairman. Glassy-eyed and tipsy, he explained that most village health committee members were away. The Chairman then dropped his polite veneer and stated in no uncertain terms that he was vexed with the Town Chief, who had not properly informed him of our visit and was not sick in bed but drunk in bed.

No health work was completed that night. Still, I did not consider the time wasted. There had been learning for the students and me.

The next day we discussed village leadership, results of Taninahun's recent community health assessment, and relationships between Serabu Hospital and the government's health centre staff.

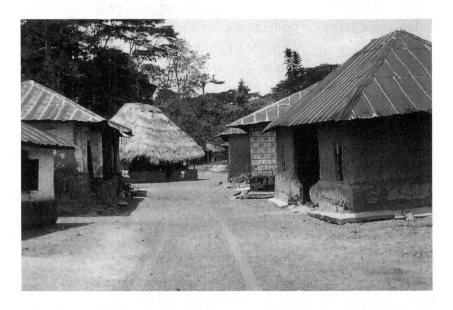

Main laterite road running through the centre of Taninahun,
a section town in Bumpe Chiefdom.

Farm Visits

When we had to locate patients on their family farms, vague directions and long treks were often involved. The search could prove futile in the end, with the patient's whereabouts unknown.

We had the names of several patients requiring follow-up in Teblahun. The village was not motorable. We parked the hospital van in Sahn and set off on a bush-path. It soon branched off. Simeon asked directions of several farmers, seeking consensus on the right path to take. Our chosen path was overgrown with scratchy grasses and thick bush; a vista of hilly terrain slowly opened up. I found the family farms indistinguishable.

We paused by a stream where a mother scrubbed laundry. Her curious, pot-bellied pre-schooler walked towards us, showing signs of malnutrition. The students gently inquired of her child's health. The woman promised to meet us in the village; we didn't see the duo again.

Serabu Hospital staff had given us the names of patients needing follow-up: a farmer who had recently been treated for a snakebite, a young man with epilepsy, the family of a baby who had died of tetanus in hospital, an older villager with suspected TB, an underweight child. It was a telling mix of cases for a small village.

The last visit of the day sticks in my mind. A 14-month-old had been seen at clinic. He had weighed in at 5.7 kg; his growth chart indicated a worrisome pattern of weight loss. His family home was vacant. An older man told us the mother had gone to her farm and gave us directions.

After a short walk, we arrived at a farm shelter. Simeon was confident we were in the right place, but no one was in sight. We called out to the mother. No answer came. We walked part-way across the farm and spotted the mother with her child. She asked us to wait in her lean-to, and soon appeared with a heavy load of rice stalks on her head, sweat glistening on her brow, and her infant dozing on her back.

We hung our portable scale from a rough beam. It added to the look and feel of obtrusion. While students weighed and examined the crying baby, his mother went about her business. She spread a mat on the ground, covered it with rice stalks, and began treading with her bare feet. We suggested treatment options for her underweight infant. The mother was adamant that hospitalization during harvest season was out of the question. We suggested a visit to the clinic the following week. She shrugged. We made feeding recommendations. She was preoccupied. I sensed that she was worried. She had been bringing her son to the clinic. Perhaps she was distressed or overwhelmed by her circumstances.

As we headed back to our vehicle, Simeon and I shared our slim hope that the mother would bring her infant for immunization. Her little one was so vulnerable to vaccine-preventable diseases.

Childhood malnutrition and *dry cough* (TB) could be a deadly mix. Malnutrition was pernicious.

I was troubled by our visit. Had we generated hopefulness or reinforced despair? Had we left the door open for a visit to the clinic or hospital? I wasn't sure. This was an out-of-the-way hamlet Serabu staff rarely visited. The villagers must have viewed us with skepticism or even dismay. Did they express doubts as to the stated reasons for our visit? Were our health messages shared? I had more questions than answers.

Flying Pigeon Bicycles

Getting to villages could be adventurous. Travel-related questions would pop into my mind as I set out with students and staff. What critters and reptiles would I encounter? Were palm-log bridges washed out? How high were the swamps? Was the hand-pulled ferry on the river operational? Would our vehicle get stuck or break down?

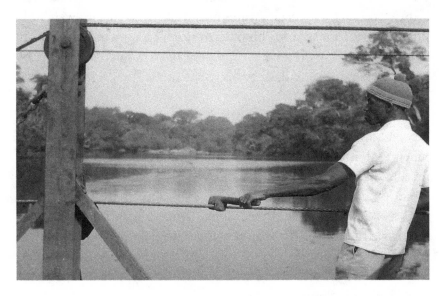

Hand-pulled ferry crossing. The boatman is wearing a touque that has been fashioned in the shape of a kufi cap.

Some travel adventures became mundane like long-jumps over marching rows of soldier ants that crossed bush-paths, or drives over three-log bridges. Others provided heart-stopping moments like the day our team crossed the fast-flowing Sewa River en route to a clinic in Sumbuya. The regular ferry was out of commission, so we clambered aboard a hired boat. Its small, outboard engine conked out as we neared the other side. Without oars, we drifted swiftly. I scanned the water for lurking crocodiles. The boatman frantically yanked on the pull cord to restart the motor, finally succeeding. Another anxiety-provoking journey under my belt.

Many travel adventures involved managing conditions outside our control. However, in a few instances, I was the primary instigator of travel problems. None more so than our fiasco with Flying Pigeon bicycles.

Our transportation needs had been growing as staff and students were deployed to more villages. Two main options had been debated. Sierra Leonean staff asserted that mopeds should be purchased, even if their cost, petrol shortages, and non-motorable villages were limiting factors. I pressed for bicycles to reach villages accessible only by bush-path. My Sierra Leonean colleagues argued that bicycles were impractical on village paths. Reluctantly, they agreed to give bikes a try.

Sister Mary ordered half a dozen Chinese-manufactured Flying Pigeon bicycles at the hardware store in Bo. I tried not to show too much enthusiasm when the bikes arrived. Paul and I planned the first bike-assisted field trip. I would take students to the village of Tungie, where we needed to identify the contacts for a TB patient who resided there. The driver would drop us off in Mokoba, and we'd cycle to Tungie. The map suggested near-perfect topographical conditions for our bike ride. Along with four students, I set off for the adventure on brand-new pedal bikes, anticipating a gangbuster day. I had something to prove.

Cycling was hard slogging. Tires dug into the sandy bush-path. We dismounted to lift our bikes over fallen trees. Crossing streams, we balanced bike wheels on narrow palm-log bridges and waded alongside. Students' faces suggested that they considered our ride on an obstacle-ridden steeplechase course to be ridiculous.

My fitness level was no match for that of my students. I was at the end of our riding pack when the track narrowed. Elephant grass suddenly towered above, slicing tiny cuts on my arms and legs. It had been a while since I'd lost sight of Edward, the student who had been directly ahead of me.

I stopped at a Y-shaped junction. Relying on my intuition and sense of direction (okay, that was not a good idea), I turned left. Panic set in. I envisioned an angry cobra rising up. I cycled faster to keep out of spitting range. I yelled out for my cycling companions. Silence.

The grass tunnel suddenly opened up to a small village. It was not Tungie. I'd taken the wrong turn. A sizable group gathered around a veranda; all eyes were cast on me. A white woman, arriving on a bicycle, who had been heard screaming in a foreign language through the long grass, made for a perplexing encounter. Youngsters ran crying into their huts, toddlers nestled into their mother's arms, and adults looked inquisitive as they tried to figure out what and who had ventured into their village. After a brief, stilted exchange involving my pathetic efforts to explain in Mende and with wild gestures who I was and why I had ridden into their village on a bicycle, I exited.

Retracing my route, I found the fork and headed off in the correct direction. Tungie wasn't much further. My students looked relieved when I showed up. They had already introduced themselves to the referred TB patient and his family. All were seated on a woven mat placed in the shade of a mango tree. I was shown to a chair. Nobody seemed interested in the specifics of my side trip.

I hoped to unravel the puzzle of TB contacts. Students interpreted. "Did either the patient or his wife have any children?"

That question was confusing to answer. "He has no *piken*, but his wife has three. Wait. Are you asking about children or grandchildren?" And then: "His wife's brothers live with them."

The spokeswoman pointed them out in the crowd—seven brothers in all. "One of them has four wives. Not all of the wives live in Tungie."

By the end of our inquiry, we had a list of 47 contacts who were dispersed across the Chiefdom. We explained the need for TB contacts to be seen at Serabu's clinic, hoping those we had met in the village would take heed. Follow-up with contacts living outside of Tungie would be near-impossible.

A crowd had gathered. Others had pressing health complaints. Two women shyly explained they could not get pregnant. I knew this was not the place to ask intimate questions about infertility.

A teenager spoke tearfully. She had a stillbirth three weeks ago and was now experiencing abdominal pain. I urged her to seek hospital treatment. Having arrived on bikes, we could not offer her a ride to the hospital even if she was ready to go.

A young man was propelled toward us—his halting gait and palsy suggested a neurological disorder. "Was this a new or old problem?" His medical history was garbled.

A lethargic and severely anemic three-year-old was brought forward, then a young infant with fever. We advised on treatment for anemia and malaria. The Chief asked an older man to stand. He had the milky eyes of river blindness. His neck and head were spotted with onchocerciasis nodules. We empathized and explained. "Doctors can't fix the blindness." We encouraged the young child beside him to continue as his seeing-guide.

Tungie was perched on the banks of the Sewa River. The older man had developed full-on river blindness. Others were harbouring the microfilia. The Sewa was a life-source for people and blackflies.

I explained that the women with infertility and the young man with the neurological disorder needed to be seen by a doctor. I was skeptical that any physician consultations would follow.

As the impromptu clinic wrapped up, women brought us a heaping bowl of *plassauce* and rice. We ate *small-small*; leftover food would not go to waste. The villagers' generosity exceeded our paltry health advice.

I turned my attention to the return bike ride. I was determined to keep up with the students. By the time we reached the van, I had conjured up another demonstration lesson. I would ride my bike all the way back to the hospital. I was pretty sure one or more students would join me for the longer biking journey. There were no takers.

Smugly, I reasoned that biking back to Serabu was an excellent chance to role model the utility of bikes on laterite roads. My decision may have been reinforced by a streak of stubbornness, since I was still on the side of demonstrating that bikes were a viable option for village work.

The pit in my stomach grew as students and driver coaxed me to change my mind. They finished loading their bikes and themselves into the van. I wavered on the inside but not on the outside. My position was firm. I waved a determined goodbye as students departed in the comfort of the vehicle. They looked more vexed than worried.

Back on my bike, I mulled over the exchange in Tungie. We had gone prepared for TB follow-up. Villagers had other health problems and created an impromptu, pop-up clinic. I felt uneasy. Had our visit raised expectations and then dashed hopes?

My pro-bike stance disintegrated as I pedalled. The slope of my bicycle seat edged backwards. The back fender rubbed against the tire. The chain was loose; the tires were soft. I still had six miles to go. What had I been thinking when I declined a ride back to Serabu?

The next village I came to was teeming with people. A ceremony to mark the death of the late Chief was underway. I was in no mood to watch the devil dancing, but I was thankful that festivities were distracting villagers' attention from me. I returned to my principled mission, now walking rather than riding my bike.

In need of a break, I stopped in Bongor to see the school's Headmaster. We awkwardly discussed first-aid kits and a latrine project for the school. He tuned out when I brought up the topic of the health committee. Perhaps the testy conversation was all on me. My attitude was sour.

As dusk fell, I arrived back in Serabu, having walked most of the way. My bike was broken and wingless. Word must have spread quickly that Miss Nancy had arrived. In class the next morning, students were wise enough to sense my bruised ego. My bike ride back to Serabu was a discussion topic temporarily off-limits. Soon, I was able to admit that I'd joined the other side of the bikes' versus mopeds' argument. My colleagues and students had been right about viable transportation options. The public health team relegated bike riding for trips in Serabu and across the hospital compound. New mopeds were ordered.

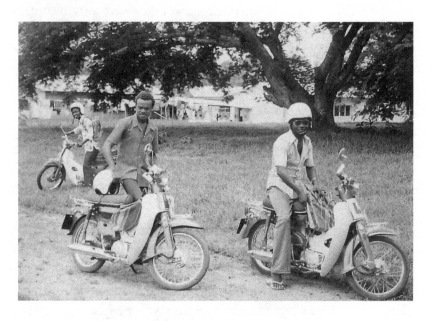

After the Flying Pigeon bicycle fiasco; mopeds for the public health team
(left to right, John, Thomas, and Simeon).

The visit to Tungie had raised other questions. Setting up, training, and supporting village health committees were our public health team's primary interventions. We risked spreading ourselves too thin when we travelled to other villages. Serabu Hospital's staff credibility could be on the line when villagers convened impromptu clinics for which we were ill-prepared. Determining what health services to offer the least accessible villages in Bumpe Chiefdom would be a recurring point of uncomfortable debate.

Stuck in the Mud

We ventured out to Sahn one evening. I was the driver for the ten-mile route. Students huddled in the back of the van. Side flaps were fastened down to keep out the heavy rain. I don't remember what we were going to do in the village that night. Our plans soon fell apart.

The bush road to Sahn consisted of a dirt track that branched off the gravel road. Bush track maintenance, which involved cutting back thick vegetation with machetes and positioning palm logs across streams, was the responsibility of each village. The status of bush roads varied tremendously. In lower-lying areas, where streams overflowed onto sandy roadbeds, maintenance was near-impossible.

Fridays were communal workdays. Villages with strong leaders generally had a better record of collaborative work. However, Chiefs were not motivated to rally men for road maintenance duties when there was no local transportation into their villages. During heavy farming season, few men had either time or energy for other work. The roadbed to Sahn had been neglected.

An eerie darkness enveloped us as I turned onto Sahn's rutted bush track. With each mucky skid, my assuredness that we would reach the village slipped away. I saw no obvious place to turn around. I tightened my grip on the steering wheel and shifted into low gear.

Three-quarters of the way into the village, the vehicle lodged in the mud. I heard a collective groan. Students gave it their best, pushing the van as I spun the wheels—forwards then backwards—sinking us deeper. Tempers frayed. I tried to hold it together. We abandoned the van and schlepped to the village to beg for a squad of men to dislodge us. The small beam of my flashlight lit our way. We arrived drenched. Everyone, except me—the incompetent driver—sported streaks and splotches of mud on their uniforms.

Croaking frogs, muted voices, and the smell of smoke from indoor fires were the only signs of life. Students located the home of the Village Chief. I explained our predicament. The Chief agreed to rouse a few men. We sheltered in the *barrie*. As each man arrived, he observed that no one else had come, stated he could not do the job alone, and after a short wait, returned home. The Chief was having one heck of a time gathering the critical mass of manpower we needed for the job. He kept at it since he would be responsible for organizing our night's lodging if the van remained stuck.

His efforts paid off. A group of tired and wiry men applied brute force and freed our vehicle. Students guided my multi-point turn. I drove the dejected team back to Serabu.

I didn't see the adventure as a *waste-time* visit. Our work had involved matters related to health, notably transportation. A sunny morning greeted us the next day. Rain had washed the heavy coating of mud off the vehicle. Once uniforms were laundered, we'd be ready to venture out to another village.

Unexpected Reactions

Health education was a constant in all of our public health work. We had key messages to convey. I wrestled with a troubling observation. Although students were good communicators when they spoke to individual families and elders, a teacher-knows-all switch turned on when they did group health education. When students reverted to lecturing, audience interest visibly waned.

We discussed the limitations of non-participatory teaching at length but students' didactic methods were well ingrained and seemed immutable. We encouraged demonstration lessons: how to cool a feverish baby, how to spoon- rather than hand-feed, and how to check for anemia. We introduced visual aids like flip charts and diagrams. Nothing seemed to break the students' rote-teaching circuit. Health messages were getting lost in the delivery process.

Furthermore, the limitations of pictorial visual aids for those with no literacy skills had become apparent. Learning to read involves making sense of words and illustrations. Children become adept at recognizing pictures through stories. We could not assume that stylized pictures or blown-up images conveyed our intended message to illiterate adults.

This realization was driven home when we tried out a portable, battery-operated slide projector in a village one evening. The students had readied a presentation on malaria. The Chief attended their health education session. On seeing the image of a mosquito on the white sheet we had hung up as a screen, he sternly told us that his village had no mosquitoes that size. Health message dismissed. That was our first and last village slide show.

We tried puppets. Connie and I spent a weekend making samples. We giggled like silly school girls as we practised an amateurish and hastily-written demonstration script, ducking behind our sofa with the puppets on stage. Although our puppet show was the first our students had ever seen, they took to the workshop, crafting puppets from basic supplies.

We had underestimated how much fun this would be, and the noise levels students would generate as they worked on their creations. Neither Connie nor I had mentioned the workshop to Sister Patricia. While we frolicked and joked, she was teaching junior nursing students new clinical skills in an adjacent classroom. Sister Patricia looked stern and shocked when she entered our class and asked us to curb the noise.

I have pictures to prove that the puppet workshop was a success. However, using puppets for health education was a flop. We tried them out with school children and then in a couple of communities. Villagers who gathered for the show looked mystified. They weren't sure what to make of the animated creatures. Youngsters ventured around the small stage to check out the student nurse puppeteers. The puppet characters were probably a source of gossip after we left, but our health messages had fallen flat. Puppets had no credibility as storytellers.

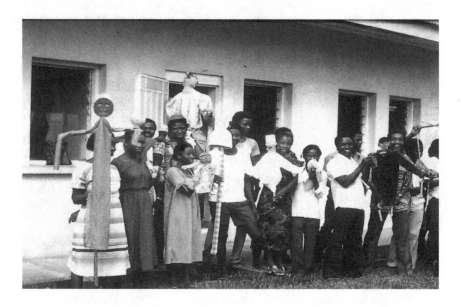

SECHN students showing off their puppet creations following workshop
(standing outside classroom on Serabu Hospital compound).

The Power of Drama

Mr. Gambai, the local Supervisor for Health Inspectors was well known for his storytelling ability. I saw him in action the evening our team arrived in Bumpe to hold a health committee meeting. Mr. Gambai was in the *barrie* sharing stories with an overflowing audience of men, women, and children. We had never had a turnout like this for a health education session, not even close.

I had heard him use parables to explain why wells, latrines, and garbage pits needed to be built. On this night, Mr. Gambai was masterful. We sat in the *barrie* with the villagers, hopeful that our meeting plans would unfold. One of my students provided whisper translation. His storytelling was riveting and suspenseful. He lightened his serious messages with humorous anecdotes.

We impatiently waited our turn, thinking the supervisor would soon be finished. He went on, and on, and on, much to the delight of his audience. We gave up. It was obvious that the village health committee had called off our meeting.

The event made an indelible impression and marked a turning point. Our public health team decided to try traditional theatre. None of us had any formal training in drama. I arranged for a dramaturg to spend a few days with us, providing guidance on the basics of script-writing and performance.[16]

Staff and students identified themes for the dramas and prepared simple storylines and character roles to convey health education messages. They performed the plays with over-the-top enthusiasm, delivering informally scripted dialogue with excellent timing. Drama was a hook. Interactive dialogue, led by the actors, followed each performance.

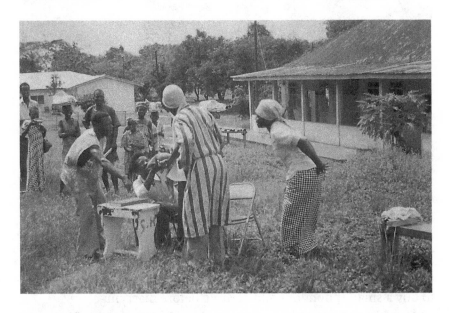

SECHN students performing a drama outside the medical ward on Serabu Hospital compound. The children's ward can be seen in background.

On arriving to perform a drama, we wove a path through the village singing familiar Mende tunes with health education lyrics. The beat of slit drums and the rattle of *segburas* drew a crowd; villagers of all ages joined in, excited by the prospect of a performance.

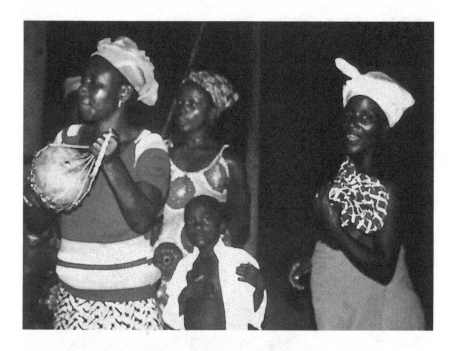

Woman playing a segbura to announce a village drama
performance by Serabu's public health team.

Each village hosted the public health drama performers as though they were part of a premier event.

Dramas were consistently met with great interest and laughter, whether students and staff performed them on the hospital grounds for mothers attending the under-five clinic or in the villages. One of our first dramas in a village concerned the risks of hand-feeding. The *barrie* was full. The Chief was engrossed and capped off a lively exchange when he pronounced that all men in his village would have to buy a small spoon for child-feeding before marrying.

One of our favourite scripts tackled hookwork anemia. The main character was a health inspector. We had earmarked the drama for a village with few latrines and conveyed our plans to the local Chief in advance.

On arriving, we were surprised and dismayed to see the local health inspector. We had tarnished relations with this gentleman, due to a clash of ideologies regarding the best way to work towards improving health conditions. We preferred a "carrot" approach (using rewards); he opted for the "stick" strategy (using punishment). He made the rounds to each village in Bumpe Chiefdom annually. This was no easy feat. The inspector's work involved many overnight stays. We did not know his schedule and rarely met him in a village. However, we heard complaints after he'd levied fines for common infractions: insufficient garbage pits, failure to dig new latrines, or general lack of cleanliness. The fines were a zero-sum game. Old habits continued, the inspector would return months later, and repeat the process.

An authoritarian health inspector repeatedly fining villagers for water and sanitation infractions was the storyline of our drama. Humour was offered at the expense of the inspector's bad character. We had two choices: reverse our plans to do the drama, thereby disappointing the community, or go ahead with the play and risk worsening our tenuous relationship with the inspector. Paul and I hesitantly opted for the latter.

Mr. Health Inspector joined the large audience. I watched him from the sidelines with trepidation. He was attentive and amused, and jumped up at the end of the drama shouting: "That's me, that's me! It's just like that! How did you know?" The inspector spontaneously took charge, leading a spirited discussion about tackling the community's endemic hookworm problem.

This was the most striking example I witnessed of the power of drama. The health inspector had a new point of connection with the community. We were relieved to have strengthened rather than fractured our relationship with him and buoyed by the villagers' suggestions for realistic sanitation improvements. Drama had opened cracks in pessimism and repositioned the cycle of fines and inaction.

CHAPTER 13
POVERTY IN THE RAW

I thought I knew poverty. Although I came from a middle-class family and grew up in a suburban neighbourhood, I had seen poverty many times. As a student nurse, I made home visits in the inner city of Windsor, Ontario. Working as a staff nurse in an emergency department, I saw the ravages of poverty among homeless patients. While a public health nurse in Newfoundland's isolated outports, I was struck by the health impacts of seasonal unemployment among fishermen.

Although I had seen poverty up close, my experiences had been more fleeting than penetrating; more intellectual than visceral. I could cite indicators that defined the class distinctions of haves and have-nots, yet I knew only superficial stories about the daily grind of being poor. My views of poverty had come through the protective lenses of a bystander, an outsider, and a clinician. I had lived apart from the poor, finding refuge in my comfortable, middle-class home and neighbourhood at the end of each work day. I had a strong inner voice about social justice, but I did not have the inner voices of those who lived poverty in the raw.

I arrived in Sierra Leone with biases and preconceptions. I had a litany of poverty assessment questions at the ready, covering matters like welfare payments, unemployment insurance, and old age security cheques. These queries were irrelevant in the villages. Sierra Leone had no social security net for subsistence farmers. Healthy children were the protective lifelines for farming families.

Not everyone in Serabu was poor. I wasn't expecting sharp class distinctions in a rural Chiefdom. The hospital staff had decent pay and lived in better-than-average homes with modest furnishings.

Their more stable financial position meant they could send all of their children to primary and secondary schools.

The local Member of Parliament had a home on the outskirts of Serabu. It stood out as a middle-class misfit with its cement blocks, glass windows, and decorative metal front door. Paramount Chiefs had more wives and owned more goats than other men. I did not think it was courteous to query their sources of income.

We occasionally met an Al Haji or Haji in the villages. Each had made a pilgrimage to Mecca and wore the elaborate religious robes demarcating this profound honour. Had their passages been paid by family members working in secure jobs in Freetown or abroad?

Foreigners who held senior positions in the nearby rutile and bauxite mines came to Serabu Hospital for care. They always arrived in a fancy car or private ambulance. If they needed to be hospitalized, they could easily afford a room in the private wing. Their payment of hospital fees offset costs waived for villagers who were admitted as charity cases.

Those from middle- and higher-income brackets were not the clientele of Serabu's primary health care program. Rather, our efforts were directed almost exclusively towards villagers living in poverty, the farmers of Bumpe Chiefdom. These were the people who enriched my understanding of what it meant to be poor. They taught me how the physical and emotional experiences of poverty ebbed and flowed with seasonal changes, and how gender and poverty were intertwined. They blew apart my erroneous belief that being poor circumscribed community character. They reshaped my health education messages and helped me understand the fragile cusp of subsistence farming.

Cycles of Poverty

Rains signalled the start of heavy and unrelenting farm labour. The work looked back-breaking; every bit was done by human hands with rudimentary tools. There were no motorized mechanical assists: no ploughs, no tractors, no harvesters, no threshers. Bumpe Chiefdom's primary landscape was tropical rain forest, a prime tsetse fly zone where animal trypanosomiasis or sleeping sickness killed draught animals. I was told that earlier efforts to introduce such livestock into the area had failed and then been abandoned.

Men began the farming season using machetes to slash trees and cut through dense growth on parcels of land that had lain fallow for seven or eight years. Controlled burning filled the air with thick smoke. White ash coated exposed earth, termite mounds, and tree stumps. When we drove through the acrid smoke of roadside farm fires, I'd nervously cover my face with my hands and a bandana, shut my eyes tight, and breathe lightly, listening for popping and crackling sounds to subside. For me, bush fires involved short bursts of exposure. For male farmers, slashing and burning was their daily work environment for a month or two, every year.

Felled trees and palm fronds were used to construct tall and sturdy A-frame shelters, where families sought refuge from the elements, cooked meals, and put little ones down for naps during long farm days. I marvelled at how quickly farm shelters were erected without winches or pulleys. The work took its toll. More men showed up in clinic complaining of back pain and muscle aches during this period of heavy labour. Accidents happened, and some injuries were life-threatening.

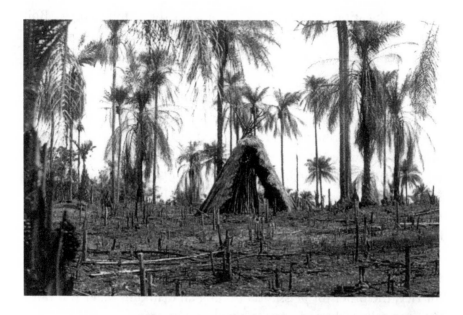

Typical A-frame shelter on upland farm.

Months of women's work followed land clearing. It looked exhausting. Women of all ages tilled the earth, inch by inch, with short-handled hoes. They planted and weeded, bent over from their waists. Verdant colours of intercropped plants poked through charcoal black. Weeds grew like they were on steroids.

When rice was nearly ready to harvest, everyone's attention turned to bird-scaring. Adults and children provided 24-hour coverage. Small elevated wooden platforms were erected. Simple noisemakers and sling-shots were used to keep weaver birds away from rice stalks. Families had little time for other matters during this taxing period of work.

Women mustered stamina for child-care duties and chores, alongside onerous farm work. As well, there was the walk from village to farm, back and forth, each day. Women carried babies and toddlers or balanced firewood on their heads. Men walked alongside, carrying foot-long machetes, as though flaunting gender inequalities.

Life was tough. It seemed impossible to lighten women's loads of day-to-day living. I squirmed with guilt. Even straight-forward health education messages could make their toil worse. Boil drinking water. Bring your children to clinic. Use a mosquito net. Feed infants pap using a cup and spoon. Not so fast—there were other considerations.

Should we ask women to boil their families' drinking water? That was a sure-proof way to decrease rates of gastroenteritis, but boiling water required firewood. Firewood had to be carried from farm to village. I consumed almost three litres of drinking water a day, more when I walked to the villages. I did the simple math. A polygamous household of ten adults required at least 30 litres of drinking water daily. That was one and a half jerry cans of water, which had to be carried from water holes to villages or farms. It was beyond unreasonable to expect women to boil that much water on three-stone fires, and in what? They had two communal household pots—one for rice, the other for *plassauce*. Boiling all drinking water was both the medically right and impossibly wrong message.

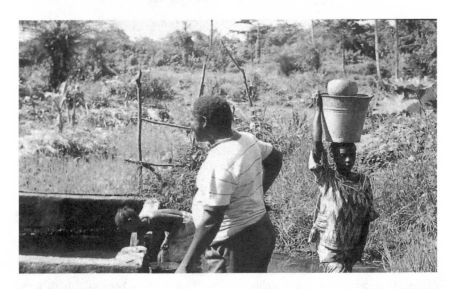

Woman and school-age girl drawing water from spring box—a semi-protected but non-potable water source. A gourd used to scoop water is floating in the woman's full bucket.

Families were advised to bring children under-five years of age to Serabu's mobile clinics, where staff monitored and advised on healthy growth and provided immunizations. Usually, mothers rather than fathers brought little ones to clinic, adding extra hours of walking to their day. Should we delay immunizations when kids were sick? This meant additional trips to the clinic.

We encouraged women to use a cup and spoon, rather than their hands, to feed an infant or toddler. This prevented overly fast hand-feeding that could result in aspiration pneumonia. I assumed basic kitchen utensils were available in every household. This was not the case. Acquiring a cup and spoon involved a cash purchase and paying for travel to a market in a larger village where such items were sold. When village women carried cash, they tied up a few coins in the corner of their *lappas*, tucking their fashioned pouches into the cloth folds around their waists. Buying market goods was not taken lightly.

Gastroenteritis could lead to acute dehydration—a medical emergency for young children. An electrolyte solution needed to be administered orally and quickly. This death-defying rehydration fluid had three ingredients: a pinch of salt, a bottle cap of sugar, and a pint-size bottle of water. Neither the measures nor the ingredients, were standard household supplies. I recall arriving in a small village where we were rushed to the home of a toddler, who was weak with dehydration, drifting in and out of consciousness in her distressed mother's lap. We asked neighbours to scour the village for salt and sugar, while the child's life hung in the balance. Electrolyte fluid was prepared. Relief grew as the toddler swallowed and sipped the fluid. Her eyelids fluttered as she regained consciousness.

As for health education messages to prevent malaria, most households could not afford bed nets. We suggested alternatives like getting rid of stagnant water near homes to discourage mosquito breeding and having chloroquine in the village so that malaria could be treated quickly.

When our public health team stuck with full-on, textbook-informed, health education messages, unfeasible advice segments derailed. Context-blind messages were rejected and spat out, undigested and indigestible.

I got mired in convoluted debates about instructions that were professionally, culturally, clinically, and contextually responsible. What health messaging was appropriate? Did health education leave mothers feeling inadequate? Did it lessen their agency? Did it leave them sensing that one more screw had been tightened in their circling cycle of poverty? No matter how well-meaning or how clearly explained, messaging that did not reflect the realities of subsistence living was, at its best, wasted effort, and at its worst, stubbornly wounding.

Drug Peddlers

Illicit salesmen who sold Western drugs acquired through the black market were a nuisance and in a class of their own. I deemed drug peddlers' tactics reprehensible. They took advantage of illiterate villagers who knew little or nothing about Western drugs' potency or side effects. Some peddlers offered *chooks* (injections) for *best price*. It was obvious when they had drummed up business. We'd see patients at clinic with festering wounds on which they had rubbed powder from a single ingestible antibiotic capsule. Mothers described having given their *piken* single, no-name pills to treat dysentery or pneumonia. Patients presented with abscesses at injection sites.

Peddlers kept a low profile and avoided Serabu Hospital staff. I guess word was out that we regarded them as a menace. Occasionally we met a brazen drug peddler in the same village where we were holding a clinic.

Our worst fear was that peddlers distributed Western medications with great potential to do harm. This was a very real possibility given their dicey drug supply sources and their limited knowledge of drugs' side effects. When word reached Serabu that a shipment of thalidomide had been stolen from Freetown's docks, alarm bells went off. The horrors of thalidomide were well known in medical circles. World-wide, over 10,000 newborns suffered congenital defects as a result of women taking that over-the-counter drug. The use of thalidomide during pregnancy had been banned. However, the drug had a redeeming feature. It was an effective treatment for an acute erythema nodosum leprosum reaction among those with Hansen's disease. While this immune response is rare, it can leave sudden, debilitating, and irreparable nerve damage. Thus, thalidomide was still on the international market.

Health professionals across the country were on high alert, fearing that unscrupulous drug peddlers might sell thalidomide as a cheap remedy for a myriad of ailments among adults, including pregnant women. We never heard reports of unusual birth defects. Maybe the stolen drugs were confiscated, or drug peddlers learned of thalidomide's terrible side effects and opted not to sell the drug.

The situation provided a stark reminder of the potential dangers of drug peddling and the particular vulnerability of those who lived in poverty. We needed to be vigilant with regard to all sources of Western medication. They were no panacea.

Seasonal Health Changes

The rains brought health woes. More children were brought to the clinic with pneumonia. Mosquitoes flourished. Rates of malaria soared and so did anemia. Groundwater run-off contaminated drinking water sources. Gastroenteritis and dehydration surged. More children had signs of acute undernutrition.

Seasonal fluctuations in childhood illnesses were often reflected on a simple graph of a child's weight against his or her age, on family-retained under-five cards. The plot was a tell-all indicator that we explained to mothers. We celebrated a robust start to life, an up-trending line showing the healthy weight gain of breastfed babies. We monitored infants as weaning foods were introduced; this was a risky period when growth often stalled, especially when it coincided with hungry season.

I was always startled by a sudden, downward shift in the growth curve. Abrupt declines in babies' growth curves required urgent attention. Plateaus or steady declines in weight over several clinic visits were worrisome.

Mothers often sensed something was amiss before weight loss was registered on a clinic scale. When inadequate growth was confirmed, mothers teared up, asking what they could do, shaking their heads when nurses' well-intentioned health education messages clashed with women's personal circumstances.

Many children did recover from acute illnesses. Mothers played their part administering medications and iron supplements, augmenting diets, and urging little ones to eat more. Some infants and children continued down a slippery slope of undernutrition. They became more passive and lethargic, lost interest in their surroundings, and lacked the energy or will to eat. In the worst cases, malnutrition seized hold, with TB as a deadly foe. Both diseases were by-products of poverty.

It gave me a sinking feeling when I looked into the listless eyes of severely underweight children. Gaunt limbs and hollowed-out faces made them look older, while their weight suggested a much younger age. With pleading expressions, their mothers sought assistance. Clinic staff tried to steer a path to recovery. Mothers urged their fragile *piken* towards wellness with soft whispers and soothing expressions of love. Hope flickered.

On rare occasions, I caught glimpse of a mother seeking to harden herself to the worst outcome, perhaps having been told by a physician or a *morie man* that her child was unlikely to survive. When malnutrition was advanced, I steeled myself for the child's demise. The pain of losses never lessened, not for public health staff and students, and especially not for mothers.

Transport Routes

Upland rice was harvested towards the end of the rains when getting produce to market was arduous. Secondary laterite roads deteriorated with incessant downpours. Low-lying areas flooded. Steep hilly routes became impassible with their exposed boulders and deep ruts—obstacles that worked in tandem to create road passage chaos. Temporary palm-log bridges laid across streams and swamps were sturdy crossing structures for creatures like lizards and rodents, but precarious for vehicles.

On the worst of these so-called roads and bridges, I behaved like a neophyte driver with my hands glued to the steering wheel as I rigidly leaned forward, and my feet did an arrhythmic quick step on clutch, gas, and brake pedals. I tried to follow hand-signalling instructions of too-anxious or overly-confident passengers acting as self-appointed guides. All the while, I anticipated the tell-tale grinding noises or lurching crunch that indicated serious trouble: a vital bit sheared off the underside or the vehicle impaled on a boulder or palm log, wheels spinning in the air.

I also experienced a passenger view of navigational challenges. Our *poda-poda* driver told riders to dismount to lighten the load. We walked behind the top-heavy vehicle; its sway exaggerated by a displaced centre of gravity. I added to the collective gasps of passengers as we watched the driver career over a so-called roadbed.

There came a point during the rainy season when even the boldest drivers concluded certain roads were too treacherous for passage. Transportation routes were cut off when palm-log bridges washed away or hand-drawn ferry crossings on rising rivers were temporarily halted. For Serabu's public health team, deteriorating road conditions were a nuisance, providing moments of heightened stress and requiring detours on a shrinking maze of still-navigable roadways. For farmers, who needed timely access to the larger food market in Bo, impassable transportation routes spelled economic disaster. And then there was the no-small-matter of the physical labour required to get produce from farm to roadside. Everything was head-carried along connecting bush-paths. The enormous exertion required to get perishable produce to roadsides could all be for naught if road transport ceased.

Never had I imagined that farm work could be so fraught with uncertainty. I had not understood the intricate links between rainy seasons and health and nutritional status, or the market difficulties of a dicey transportation network. My regard for the skills and tenacity of farm families had doubled with my own failed gardening efforts, and then mega-tupled as I experienced seasonal growing cycles and transportation challenges. Farmers could do little to make the difference between a hungry or a hungrier season.

Food Supply Chains

The food supply chain was not an abstract, textbook concept. It was not hidden behind the consumer-oriented interface I knew in Canada with its grocery chains, shelves of canned goods, rows of refrigerators replenished with dairy and meat products, and advertising flyers. In Serabu, each weak link in the local food chain was visible: scarce market foods, a rise in the cost of staples, less protein added to *plassauce*. Villagers teetered between food security and insecurity.

Bumpe Chiefdom seemed far removed from distorting industrial players in food production and distribution. Conglomerate mega-farms were being developed in other areas, and I pondered their encroachment. Did agricultural inroads provide the economic boost needed to bring better health and education services to the people? That was the stated goal of agricultural development projects. In fleeting drives alongside the palm oil plantations that dotted the countryside near Freetown, I saw no evidence of better housing or infrastructure in nearby villages. I wondered who the primary beneficiaries of mega-farms were.

Plantations were leaving a topographic dent—or was it a scar—on the landscape. Sun piercing through neatly ordered rows of trees created unnatural geometric patterns of light on the ground; a striking contrast to the diffuse light of dense tropical rain forests. Large-scale plantations looked ecologically fraught. Their imposed order uncannily distorted nature's disorder.

I got an up-close look at palm oil plantations near Mile 91. This is where the Magbosi Integrated Agricultural Development Project was operating. Economic development was its primary thrust. The initiative also aimed to improve health. I joined Simeon Sisay, a Sierra Leonean agricultural economist, to oversee an assessment of 250 households that would provide baseline measures of villagers' health and nutrition status. A group of Serabu's community health nursing students conducted the interviews. Health status was even worse than in Bumpe Chiefdom.[17]

During village interviews, I heard troubling stories of the disruptive, local impact of cash crop development. Villagers described swamps that had permanently dried up, eliminating women's dry season vegetable plots. Plantations held the promise of future benefits. Women asked how to feed their children today. Their stories laid bare the challenges of agricultural economic development. Palm oil harvests could augment profit margins, but for whom, at what cost, and in what timeframe?

Agricultural projects had winners and losers. The villagers' pointed questions left me skeptical about the promised trickle-down benefits of new mega-farms for the poorest villagers. Little ones might not survive the immediate consequences of cash-crop-induced malnutrition. Health could be seriously threatened by fraught paths to development.

Ribs of Poverty

Poverty had to be taken into account in everything we did because it was everywhere and implicated everyone. I began to understand the local experiences of poverty. I reshaped health messages to minimalist and shaky economic realities. I gained a new appreciation of other sectors implicated in health improvements. And then I had a disturbing realization. It dawned on me that, for the most part, I was working within—rather than on—the roots of poverty. I was not a citizen of the country. I had no direct links to the levers of government, either traditional or parliamentary. CUSO had an unwritten rule for volunteers to be apolitical. Big "P" (policy) advocacy was out of the question. I questioned my role as a change agent.

I reassured myself. Little "p" advocacy was infused in our public health work. We used a nudge strategy in the villages. We got the support of Chiefs for TB control plans and immunization campaigns. We asked TBAs to urge the husbands of high-risk pregnant women to allow their wives to go to hospital for delivery. We persuaded traditional healers to have chloroquine tablets available for the treatment of malaria. We dispelled complacency; the status quo was not acceptable.

At times my thinking about small "p" advocacy work verged on grandiose. I boldly told Serabu's public health team and students that if President Siaka Stevens understood what our primary health care activities were fostering in Bumpe Chiefdom, he would be concerned by our activism. Village by village, we were beginning to reshape expectations of health and health services, and seeding a different future, particularly for women and children. Small successes gave me goosebumps. Still, I had moments of sober reflection. How would I know if our advocacy had gone far enough? Was there a tipping point for raised village expectations that fostered malcontent? Traditional leaders provided a buffering interface, course correcting over-zealous advocacy by Serabu's public health nurses.

Inner Guiding Voices

Slowly, villagers I met were becoming my inner voices. Their stories and circumstances gave poverty personality, shape, and texture. Their narratives of hope, perseverance, advocacy, fortitude, and anguish were starting to reside within me.

Mansaray, the shy, but staunch advocate for her four youngsters. She had reached out to our public health team when we visited Blama.

Isatu and other TBAs, who proudly shared stories of the midwifery services they had provided for decades. They actively recruited younger women to this work, recognizing the importance of capacity renewal. They soaked up the content of lessons to provide better care.

The mother who shook with anguish as her infant lay dying of tetanus in her arms. Her sobs still echo in my psyche. I hear her pleading for her baby, for all newborns, for every mother. *Soin-soin* should not take our little ones.

Families who knew something was amiss with an initiative that brought the economic promise of cash crops while wiping out self-reliant dry season vegetable plots. Their intimate connection to the land laid bare unintended consequences of a development project.

Fodia, the little girl who befriended me in Serabu. Her farming family was poor, dirt-poor. I loved Fodia's innocence, her joie de vivre, her pride. I have a nagging question. Did Fodia have the opportunity to get an education? I regret not asking her mother about schooling for her daughter.

The omnipresence of poverty filled Serabu's public health team with determination, while keeping us grounded in the day-to-day realities of being poor. It united us in creative endeavours to deliver culturally-relevant public health services. Our primary health care efforts mattered; change for the better was possible. New inner voices and images of poverty in the raw took hold in my conscience.

CHAPTER 14
WITCHES

"Let the witch people no humbug you," was the Town Chief's affable greeting. He wished no harm or ill will to befall Serabu's public health team. His expression reflected a vital and preoccupying truth. Witches could wreak much havoc, illness, and instability. The wrath of witches was to be avoided at all costs.

Beliefs in witches were ubiquitous among the Mende. If not witches, what other explanation could there be for unfortunate ills? Why did some farmers have crop failures, while other farms thrived in the same rainy season? How was it that the dreaded *nyenye* took the lives of *piken* one year but not another? Why wouldn't a witch be the explanation for serious social transgressions? Wasn't this a warning from the ancestors?

Tackling witches required the heavy duty know-how and expertise of *morie men* and sorcerers. These traditional healers were steeped in the ways of witches. They advised on the messy business of witch-induced circumstances and questions. Should a witch hunter be called? Could a witch be driven from the village? Where did one's allegiance fall when a family member was accused of being a witch?

Witches were mean-spirited. They ravaged all facets of life. To protect upland farms, *jujus* were buried on the main paths leading to a farm hut. Above-ground *jujus* were common, although initially out of my perceptual gaze. Mende colleagues pointed them out as we walked past farms: stones, sticks, and strings arranged so as to catch or scare away a lingering witch or bad spirit. *Jujus* made of cloth and string were visible on the exterior of some homes.

Villagers tried to navigate around witches to instill social harmony and show respect for ancestors. Beliefs in sorcery defined taboos and guided functions like where women should draw water, bathe, and fish. Ancestors were vital to community integrity. Their powers were pseudo-antidotes to witchcraft.

Many illnesses were believed to be caused by witches. I was perplexed by a Mende term I heard at my first immunization clinic. As nursing students explained the purpose of *marcleates* (immunizations) to mothers, they used a modified English word, *germsie*. Students said there was no word for "germ" in the Mende language. I asked: "What did mothers believe caused common childhood illnesses?"

The students' responses were swift and detailed. *Nyenye* was caused by a witch spraying hot water on a child at night, thus producing the red rash and fever. Polio (*indele*) resulted when a boa constrictor partially swallowed a child at night. Boas were thought to be witches, harboured by widows or widowers who sought companionship now that their spouse was gone.

Since the term *germsie* was meaningless, we changed our description of how immunizations protect a child. "The *marcleate* helps a child fight the witch who causes the disease."

Rightly or wrongly, Paul and I determined that locally informed, rather than biologically construed terminology, was a more effective way to encourage women to bring their children for immunization. I supposed my microbiology professors would be appalled with our explanations.

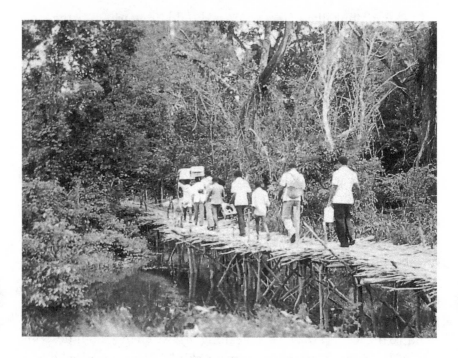

*Public health team and SECHN students carrying vaccines
and supplies to village immunization clinic.*

Burial Practices

The presence, and thus necessary avoidance, of witches in villages was pervasive. When a death was suspected to have been caused by a witch, burial practices had to be adjusted accordingly. Squatting on stools in the *Bundu* bush on the outskirts of a small village, TBAs explained this to me through their animated exchange. A female student translated.

Journal Entry

October 24th, 1980

The midwives spoke in excited voices. They were very intent on explaining the witch business to us, talking all at once and emphasizing their stories with gestures. They explained the havoc created by witches and the practices TBAs used to reduce the potential for more harm. The *Sowei* began:

> A woman in obstructed labor will sometimes confess that she has a witch. It is believed that if she does [have a witch], she and/or her baby will die. Nobody can do anything to prevent this. When she dies, she is buried far from the town. Rice is left between the graves of mother and baby. No woman is ever allowed to pass near this burial place.

She went on to explain that this prohibition protected other women and their children from being harmed by the witch.

In the same sitting, these TBAs related an astounding story:

> In another village, a woman confessed to being a witch. Many children had died in that village that year. The woman said that she had consumed 50 children. Her own baby died following childbirth. Another woman had a dream in which she saw all the children who had died—one of the dead children had come to take this witch. The woman related the dream to a friend the next morning. Wailing was then heard from the home where the woman who was possessed by the witch had just died.

Since a witch was capable of entering a pregnant woman and harbouring in her womb, special precautions were taken after a woman died in labour. TBAs removed the fetus from the mother's body and buried it separately to reduce chances of the offending witch bringing harm to other villagers. Some traditional midwives had seen the internal reproductive anatomy of women, having conducted postmortems as part of burial practices.

Families blamed witches for illnesses and deaths, especially among children and child-bearing women. The aftermath of witchcraft often played out for years. In a remote village, a middle-aged man told me that his three children died of fever and his wife died because of witchcraft in the wife's family.

One day I dreamt people were killing an animal in my home. In the morning, I explained this to the elders, and they told me it was witchcraft either in my family or my woman's family. My wife was pregnant by then. After a month, she was admitted to hospital where she delivered a premature baby. After two days, the child died. After a week, my wife died. I went to a native sorcerer, and he told me it was the work of witchcraft. I then decided to marry another woman who is not staying with me. She has no children. I still feel [that] the witchcraft of my late wife is playing evil with my family.

Witch stories left me shaken and a little less certain that I was a non-believer. A gradual shift in my thinking started to take shape. My early inclination had been to deny and argue against the plausibility of witches. During mass immunization campaigns, invoking such arguments had proven linguistically impossible and counterproductive. Besides, older people were enthusiastic about immunizations, having seen the eradication of smallpox in their lifetime, and although not vaccine-related (but it did involve injections of penicillin), the near-elimination of the highly contagious yaws. Elders expressed their strong support for immunizations. Did it matter that they had a different belief system than I or other Western-trained health providers at the hospital?

Nursing students were not troubled by the duality of their beliefs. On one hand, they could describe the microbiology of common infectious diseases. Students had seen disease pathogens (bacteria, protozoa, and amoeba) under a microscope. They knew the life cycle of common infectious diseases and were staunch supporters of vaccine campaigns. On the other hand, all of my students believed in witches and cited proof of their existence.

My arguments for exclusively non-witch causal agents were defeated when I required an appendectomy during my fourth year in the country. I had no satisfactory answer for my students who asked: "What witch had put the germs in my abdomen that caused my appendicitis?"

Possibly, I too had had the misfortune of invoking the wrath of a witch. When, where, and how, I'll never know.

Kemamoi

In the midst of a crisis, a community might decide to identify the person who was harbouring the witch or using witchcraft and then *drive the witch* from the village. This meant that the individual(s) implicated was forced to leave and seek refuge in another community. This was serious punishment and made them social outcasts. I judged it overly harsh with the potential to scapegoat. But then, lives were at stake, and the health of other villagers hung in the balance.

The practice of banishing witches was highly problematic for villagers who had a contagious disease like TB. Their movement from one village to another increased the risk of transmitting TB and made thorough case-finding efforts unworkable.

When the devastating consequences of witches' work were seen to be at play, communities sometimes hired *kemamoi*. These sorcerers had special powers to identify witches. One night, we headed out to a village where a dreadful epidemic of measles was still taking children's lives. This super-spreader contagion led the Village Chief to call in the *kemamoi*. The *barrie* was bursting with people. Along with my public health colleagues, I was spellbound by the ceremonies that were taking place in an area cordoned off by locally spun cotton strings. There seemed no alternate explanation(s) for the outcome of rituals performed, all aimed at locating the witch. Witch-believer or not, who was I to question the importance of invoking the power of a witch finder to prevent further illness and restore health to a village?

Experiences with *kemamoi* reinforced convictions that witches were at fault. An epidemic of measles, gastroenteritis, or whooping cough would come to the end of its natural course around the same time that the witch pegged as responsible for the outbreak was forced to leave the village.

The community's preoccupation with witches sometimes slowed or derailed public health work. Yet, the community's tactics to weaken the power of witches were part of, rather than apart from, this work. In a 1981 document summarizing bi-annual progress with health committees in ten villages not too far from Serabu Hospital, the work of witch hunters was frequently described. A constellation of problems had led villagers to seek their services.

Foya, with a population of 510, was a section village several miles from the Chiefdom headquarters. It had been the site of vaccination clinics and was participating in the World Food Program.

> Foya recently hired a witch hunter, feeling that it was not finding its fair share of diamonds, too many children were dying, and successful people were not returning to the town to retire. The [witch hunter's] accusations have created antagonisms that are making full cooperation in primary care projects difficult at present.[18]

Walihun, a village of 1066, had frequent visits from Serabu's public health team. They too had hired a witch hunter.

> Walihun's inhabitants were concerned that successful people are not returning to retire in the village, the [small] plantations are not successful, there is too much TB [eight sputum-diagnosed TB patients lived in the village—four others had died and three had left the town in the last six months]. Too many children are dying and the shopkeepers are not staying...The [community's] preoccupation with witch-finding proceedings has slowed down primary care activities.[19]

Regardless of my own incredulity about witches and *kemamoi*, these entities were a big part of Mende life and could not be ignored. This was not a case of Western ideas being right and traditional beliefs being wrong. The essence of our work was to identify common touch points that unleashed the joined-up strengths and strategies of Serabu's public health team and villagers. I concluded that belief systems do not need to be compatible for the pursuit of complementary efforts.

I came to understand that witches represented far more than a disbelief in biological pathogens. Explanations of witches at work were not a simple replacement for notions of disease causation. Rather, they concerned larger social circumstances: poverty, vulnerability, and insecurity. Harmonious living was necessary for survival among interdependent farmers. The presence of a witch was a source of disharmony and a potential threat to everyone's well-being. Averting, identifying, and *driving witches* from villages were essential preventive and restorative public health strategies.

CHAPTER 15

How deh go, deh go?

Village health committees were the heart of Serabu's primary health care approach. By the late 1970s, the program had grown from three pilot villages to eleven communities. We wanted to better understand the guts of health committee work. In 1980, Sister Hilary announced it was time for a circuit tour to probe the experiences of committee members. We had questions. How did the committees function? What were their successes and difficulties? What supports did they need? What matters were starting to seethe? Frank dialogues with Chiefs and committee members would guide course corrections.

Committee members were keen to meet directly with Mama Hilary. She was the big chief, the boss, and the head honcho for Serabu's public health team. With other demands on her time, Sister Hilary rarely did this kind of village outreach. She intervened when a crisis occurred. A major palaver. A health calamity.

Sista Docta Hilary's presence would bring an element of gravitas to the dialogue with village health committees. Public health staff, who provided monthly supervisory support for committees, anticipated Sister Hilary's back-up reinforcement of their efforts. Mama Hilary was well known for her humorous storytelling antics. She could make anyone laugh. Her potential entertainment value would encourage attendance. We hoped for onlookers, as the dialogue would profile committee members.

I was eager to hear members describe their experiences as a collective. In day-to-day work, we met with members individually, providing tailored training sessions or sorting-out issues pertinent to their specific responsibilities. The planned visits would allow us to *hang heads* (consult and dialogue) in the Mende way.

Alongside the local Chief, Sister Hilary took the lead for each meeting. She tried to keep her questions and explanations pointed and crisp. Paul translated, English to Mende, and Mende to English.

My job was to offer Sister Hilary prompts and background information or points of clarification. Students took notes. I captured excerpts of what was said and what my students heard from bystanders. In the margins of my notebook, I recorded impressions.

En route back to Serabu, the team reflected on what we'd learned. I wished to be a fly on the wall to hear the parallel, debriefing conversations in the village.

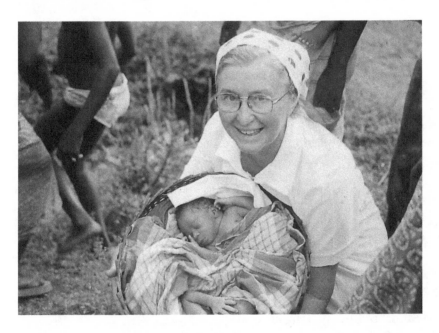

Newborn twins had been delivered by a TBA just a few hours before we spotted them being carried on a path alongside the road. Basket with twins held by Sister Hilary Lyons.

Village Health Committees: Community Consultations

Journal Entries

October and November 1980

Bangor

The *barrie* has been prepared with bush lamps, a couple of small wooden tables, and rickety chairs. Members of the health committee explain their work.

"The medicine man is a farmer; he is quite well known for his knowledge of herbal medicine."

Sister Hilary encourages him. "Continue learning this trade from the old Pa [the older native medicine man in the village] before all is forgotten."

The Chief requests "new learning so they may improve health of the town."

The man responsible for sanitation proudly states: "Twenty-four compost fences have been constructed. The town needs teaching for their proper use."

A torrential rainstorm begins. The downpour on the *barrie's* zinc pan roof is deafening. Committee members' voices are drowned out. I strain to hear the translation. The formal meeting is cut short but many hang around.

We are taken aside by a traditional midwife. A female nursing student translates. "She learned midwifery from her mother-in-law. She is part-Hausa."

I try not to stare at the long and prominent scarification on her cheeks. She shares her family history.

"Her father was a sheep farmer. He travelled to Nigeria, and there he met the Hausa woman who became his wife." She begins explaining her midwifery work emphasizing, "She does not receive any payments for deliveries. She stays in her village at all times in case a woman goes into labour."

Her statement does not ring true. This is a farming community; there are not enough births to keep her busy all the time. I wonder why she is being so guarded about her role as a midwife. It's unusual for a TBA to set herself apart from other granny midwives in the community. Given her mixed heritage, I wonder if she is a member of the *Bundu* Society and accepted by the other traditional midwives.

A few pregnant women are listening to the exchange with this Hausa woman; quiet side conversations are taking place among them.

Later, the students tell me these women had explained: "They must *put small* (pay) for a delivery, with rice, a chicken, and money."

There's a social disconnect here, but I've hardly scratched the surface. Every bit of questioning and explanation has to be translated. I avoid digging too deep; it's impossible to get the full story.

As we stand up to leave, Munda rushes up to the veranda where we're saying our good-byes to the Chief. Munda greets our team, a big smile on his face. We all recognize the scrawny and unkempt ten-year-old. This year he's already had two episodes of hospitalization in Serabu's children's ward, following grand-mal epileptic seizures that resulted in burn injuries when he fell onto hot coals. Munda is in the care of his grandmother. She is very old and forgets to give Munda his phenobarbital. It has been difficult to get Munda to assume more responsibility for taking his medication regularly.

When this pre-teen was last discharged, he told the nurses that he wanted to return to the children's ward because he preferred to live there. It's a sad situation. There are no youth or child protection services to intervene, no social workers to call on. I am worried Munda will ask us to take him back to Serabu when we leave. He does not. I hope this means he is more content to be staying with his grandmother.

Sahn

Tonight, the road to the village is very bad. It's narrow and bushy with trenches that jostle us in the van. I'm relieved that Lansana, "PHD", as he calls himself, is at the wheel. His self-proclaimed "PHD" stands for public health driver. Lansana navigates the track slowly and safely.

The Chief is praying at the mosque. While awaiting him, we visit a 13-year-old TB patient. She has not been taking her medicine as instructed. Sister Hilary calls a family meeting. A couple of adults slump in hammocks; others perch on small stools. Four young school-age children lean in curiously to hear the exchange. Sister Hilary explains the importance of thiazine. Adults nod in agreement. I wonder what they're thinking. The teen leans awkwardly against a veranda post, staring at the ground while we discuss her TB medication compliance. Patient confidentiality as I know it, doesn't exist in these close-knit villages.

We move back to the *barrie*. Bystanders join. The meeting quickly turns into an attack session regarding logistics. It's not a good start.

In response to a question from Sister Hilary about public health visits, the Chief states, "There is no problem with the nurses coming to Sahn. They are happy to receive the nurses."

The headwoman has a complaint. "When they cook for our team, the nurses refuse to eat the food, stating it is not good enough for them." Sister Hilary and Paul query this assertion. It's difficult to get a straight story.

With prompting from Paul, Sister Hilary asks "What happened to the letter we sent five months ago about unsatisfactory conditions for the nurses? We have received no reply."

The Chief begs forgiveness. He changes the topic and raises questions about the four well sites selected last year. No progress has been made. He asks when Serabu's public health team will initiate well construction. There's a misunderstanding. Constructing the well is the village's responsibility. The health committee wants to write us a letter stating what they want done and what they'll do for Serabu's nurses. There is an undercurrent of dependence on handouts.

Riding back to Serabu, we share our thoughts. I found the meeting discouraging.

Paul comments on self-sufficiency. "I would like to take one small village. I would explain that Serabu Hospital will give them nothing. They must do things for themselves. We would help with learning."

"Isn't this what we're already doing?" I ask.

Paul explains, "We may have created unrealistic expectations in Sahn." He cites the example of Yengima, "where they have been constructing a home for the nurse over the past four years and erroneously expect it to be staffed by a Serabu Hospital nurse when it's built."

Student nurses overheard people saying that bad things shouldn't be discussed with the white people present. They seem to be afraid of losing our services.

John suggests, "We should have a health committee from one of the three pilot villages visit Sahn to explain their functions."

Always, there are new problems. It's difficult to see around the obstacles. The expressions heard tonight included "these people" and "in our culture". We agree this is human nature—change is slow in all of us.

As we drive into Serabu, Thomas exclaims that electricity has come to the village. An area of town that is far from the hospital compound appears to be illuminated. We all laugh. The headlights of a lorry are reflecting off a white-washed home. We too, have had our expectations dashed. What seems, may not be.

Mokoba

Despite the heavy rain, there is a good turnout of health committee members. We're uncomfortably seated on low, wobbly benches inside the primary school. Insects buzz around the bush lamps. Remnants of an arithmetic lesson are on the rough chalkboard.

The Section Chief, Acting Town Chief, and school's Headmaster are present. Committee members are invited to describe their roles. One by one, they do so, pretty much parroting what's in their role description.

I like the explanation provided by the agriculture man. "He is responsible for assessing adequate food production because food is essential for health. Medicine does no good if there is no food."

The Chairman raises the village's request for a clinic. The TBA signals her agreement.

The Chief is on board. "A clinic would be well attended by those from surrounding villages, including the villages of Sembehun-Tabe (Tikonko Chiefdom) and Verima (Lugbu Chiefdom)."

The woman responsible for under-five children chimes in. "The health committee will have responsibility for the clinic as long as the Chiefs support them and give them small power."

The Section Chief nods approvingly. "All members of the health committee will be involved with a clinic—the agriculture man, everyone."

Sister Hilary explains: "It is necessary for them to learn a basic set of lessons first."

Their response is enthusiastic. "They will lodge a nurse for a week so the lessons can be taught. Feeding is not a problem—there is much rice in the village now, the result of swamp rice development this year."

Sister Hilary presses them for other health priorities.

The Chief indicates they "will decide on other activities for the coming year like building latrines and a water well."

Their unanimity suggests they considered these matters beforehand. I hope their enthusiasm lasts.

Mokpendeh

After greeting the Chief, we try to meet with the Al Haji. With her elaborate and voluminous head tie, she's easy to spot. She gives us a cool reception and acts like she was not expecting us. Sitting on a small stool, she has bunched-up her long gown in her lap, while she toilet-trains her granddaughter. The child squats, her chubby thighs supported by the grandmother's feet, the toddler's bare bum near the ground. "Woosh, woosh," her grandmother whispers, urging her grandchild to void. She is on child-care duty; too preoccupied to join tonight's event.

We make our way to the *barrie*. Numerous health committee members are in attendance, as well as interested onlookers. The Chief arrives, welcomes our team to the village, and invites us to begin.

Sister Hilary stands up and asks the committee to tell us about their health.

The Section Chief asserts, "It is rainy season, so things are difficult for us."

Sister Hilary nods with empathy. She continues: "What is the main thing needed for a *well body*?"

"Farming" is the truncated translation of the Chief's serious response. This is the answer I've often heard to one of Sister Hilary's favourite questions. Being dependent on the land, farmers understand the tethered link between crop yields and health.

Health education and medicine are mentioned as benefits of nurses' visits. The Chief makes a new request: "Now we want a well to prevent diarrhea and vomiting because some people are passing stool upstream."

Sister Hilary probes: "What other sicknesses do they get?"

Health committee members chime in. "Headache, eye problems, and river blindness among adults. Fever, rashes, tetanus, scabies, and ringworm among children."

The woman responsible for under-five children enthusiastically leans in, "Measles is better now." Her response triggers rapid banter among committee members.

Paul explains. "They disagree about the reason. The men say it's because of the rainy season; the women say it's due to immunizations."

Sister Hilary continues, "Does the committee meet regularly?"

The response is negative; no explanation is offered. The Chief looks uncomfortable. The committee chair breaks the silence. "We want nurses to come and stay with us for a week to teach us. We want to start lessons in dry season."

Sister Hilary isn't going to wait until dry season to insert a short TB lesson. She describes how people get the disease and how to prevent it. She emphasizes the take-home message. "Treatment takes at least one year with medicine."

The Chief has been listening attentively. He responds, "There is a man in town who is getting native medicine for *dry cough*. I will present him at the next village health committee meeting."

My mind wanders. I wonder what "presenting him" to the committee involves. Will such an act of public disclosure move this man any closer to getting the Western treatment he needs? With the influx of artisanal miners to Mokpendeh, an active case of TB is worrisome. Their living conditions are crowded.

Sister Hilary moves onto another topic. "I know Mokpendeh is not an easy town because people come and go."

The Chief quickly asserts. "Lack of unity is a big problem. It is worse in the dry season when many Temne come to mine diamonds."

One health committee member is cynical. "If nurses were sent to give health education to Temne families, when those mothers leave, that will be the end of it." There are obvious tensions between the permanent residents and temporary visitors from other villages and tribes.

The Chief changes the topic. "He still wants the nurses to come and assist them to improve sanitation."

Sister Hilary is firm. "The village should take the responsibility of feeding the nurses when they come." She invites the Temne to speak for themselves. "Do those from the Temne tribe have any questions?"

Their spokesperson hesitantly steps forward and responds quietly in Mende, "The Temne are foreigners here and always cooperative."

Sister Hilary offers final words. "The public health team will come back with vaccines for immunization. Villagers will need to bring their *piken* to the clinic. It is up to them to make the effort."

The Chief gives a parting response. "He wants us to continue coming and to be patient with them."

On the ride home, I recall a prior conversation. Our public health team had been told that men have to sleep in shifts during diamond mining season to accommodate the influx of male miners. We've been concerned about potentially high rates of sexually transmitted diseases but these weren't on their list of health issues. I should have discussed this with Sister Hilary beforehand. I don't know if this topic needs to be addressed separately with men and women. I've been in the country for two years, and I'm still a communication neophyte. There are endless cultural nuances I don't understand when it comes to sexual health matters.

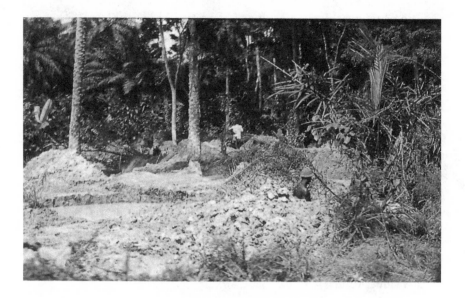

Alluvial diamond mining and miners near Mokpendeh, Bumpe Chiefdom.

Walihun

Paul and I notify the Section Chief of our arrival while Sister Hilary goes off to speak to the private dispenser about TB drugs. There are active TB cases in Walihun; some are defaulting on their treatment protocols despite being close to Serabu. Sister Hilary wants to bring the dispenser on board so that he too will encourage TB patients to comply with their treatment.

We're dismayed when the Chief indicates he failed to notify others of the event. The Chairman is away for a burial, and the clerk is holding a meeting of churchgoers. Noting our reaction, the Chief hurriedly instructs a young man to call households by hitting the piece of metal used as a school bell and blowing an animal horn. The noises are loud enough to reach the distant huts up on the hillside.

We gather in the *barrie* as villagers arrive. Small benches have been arranged inquisition-style; the white *pomweis* (myself included) and Serabu Hospital nurses in a single row, facing health committee members and the Chief. A mixed crowd looks on from the sidelines. At the Chief's request, each committee member stands up in front of us as they describe their roles.

Sister Hilary cuts through the uncomfortable formality asking, "*How deh go, deh go?*"

The Chief responds with confidence, "Since the health committee was formed, measles and tetanus have almost finished. They are pleased that children have received BCG vaccinations. They are planning to *drive out* TB patients from their town who are refusing to take treatment. They plan to inform the Paramount Chief of this decision tomorrow."

I'm skeptical. The timing is too coincidental. They know Sister Hilary is trying to clamp down on TB defaulters. There's a hint of appeasing Mama Hilary with their planned action that does not reassure. *Driving* TB patients away spreads the disease to other villages.

The Chief turns to other matters. He reports that the maternity home, which they started to build months ago, "is finished." It's a qualified version of finished. "The Chief is asking for help to complete the home."

The committee's Chairman indicates "they want help improving their water source."

The sanitation man pipes in and lists diseases villagers can get from contaminated drinking water: "diarrhea, dysentery, abdominal distension. These are really bad for children."

Other committee members nod in agreement. The Chairman puts forward suggestions. "They would like the list of lessons they have been taught. If the nurses stopped coming, they would continue to do what they have learned improves health. If immunization stopped, they'd come to Serabu to ask why."

Sister Hilary smiles and explains she is pleased to hear this. "You pay hut taxes and have the right to immunization. Serabu Hospital does not get any of the hut tax revenue." This is an important clarification although I think the intent of Sister's message about health care funding is lost.

The sanitation man turns the dialogue back to matters of potable water and latrines. "They'd like our help. They need a well digger. Where are we to get such a person?"

Sister Hilary explains. "I have contacts."

The Chief provides operational details. "Villagers will dig the well, but they need financial help for cement and a well pump." Smiling, he comments on Sister's expertise. "We know Sister Hilary digs in stomachs, not wells."

Sister Hilary responds, "I'd like to put fire in the committee members so they are not always asking for handouts." A wave of chuckles ripples among committee members. I think they've heard her say that before.

The agriculture man on the committee brings up a related matter. "Our coffee crop is not good this year; there has been too much sun. We have less money from this cash crop."

Sister asks, "Did they contact the agricultural technician?"

Committee members deny knowing the technician.

Sister encourages them to be proactive and independent. "God sent you the agricultural technician; you should go to him."

The Chief responds with a local reality check. "Times are getting harder. Even when we try, it is still difficult."

Sister Hilary nods with understanding. She broaches a new topic. "How can the committee transfer their knowledge to others in the town?"

The Chief has suggestions. "Each village section is represented by one committee member. When each committee member goes home, he/she should gather a group of people and explain the health lessons to them. Most of their health committee members have deputies."

The Chief has pondered this question of outreach.

I prompt Sister Hilary to ask about the dramas we've been doing in villages, including Walihun. She asks, "What do they think of the dramas?"

The Chief responds. "If we had a drama tonight, we would have had many more people come."

Committee members are suddenly animated, chatting among themselves. The Chairman speaks. "The committee members want to take part in a drama. With practice, we could learn our parts." Smiles and clapping all-around. I'm heartened by this enthusiasm for traditional theatre.

Sister Hilary returns to more mundane business. Her questions about record keeping are for the clerk.

Paul translates with a hint of cynicism in his voice. "The clerk is not keeping a record of birth and deaths because the people don't come to him."

Sister Hilary reminds the clerk, "Recording births and deaths is very important. Unless we know how many children are born and die, we don't know if the committee is effective or not."

The clerk looks down, offering no response. I wonder whether and how he understands the notion of effectiveness. We use that term a lot in our public health lingo. I make a mental note to ask Paul if there is a direct translation for the word "effectiveness" in Mende.

The child-care worker confidently answers Sister Hilary's questions about nutritious food and immunizations. Sister Hilary praises her. "She has done her job well. She helps with the under-five clinic. The public health team is grateful for her contributions."

"Do you have a good native medicine man?" Sister Hilary inquires.

The Chief takes that question. "There is a good one in their town for children. He has medicine for convulsions."

One of the committee members snickers at the Chief's response and explains the irony of the situation. "People trust more in the hospital now. The hospital took away the native healer's business. So it is difficult for him to earn a living."

I wonder if this is a good or bad thing. Either way, it's an unintended consequence of having set up a village health committee in Walihun.

Kpetema

We arrive in the midst of Muslim prayers and wait in the prepared *barrie*. We are each lost in our thoughts.

Health committee members start to arrive, slowly taking their seats. Quiet conversations are taking place when Mr. Chala, the Headmaster, bursts onto the scene. He authoritatively gets right into business, abrasively stating in English, "I want to find out who are the non-attenders of the meeting."

I'm taken aback by his chastening remarks. Committee members seem nonplussed. I think he's making a show of his authority.

I'm distracted by the background chatter of children playing under a full moon. They soften the scene as Sister Hilary begins with her first question. "How do they see the health committee business?"

The Section Chief responds. "They used to get plenty of *sick*, which they no longer have." I suspect they are telling us what they think we want to hear.

Sister Hilary presses for more information. "Is the committee a help or a *humbug*? Is the committee still on the right road?"

A spokesperson for the committee explains, "They think it's a very good thing and want to continue. Previously, the sanitary overseer came every few months to fine them. The committee has now understood why it is important to scrape the grass, daub their homes, and protect their water source."

Senasie, the sanitation man, stands up and describes his duties as "instructing people to scrape, brush, and improve water supplies and latrines." There is pride in his mannerisms and voice as he explains, "The villagers have now understood the importance of latrines; they're digging them with his instructions. They now have garbage disposal areas."

Sister Hilary indicates she is pleased with the committee's progress on sanitation.

The committee's Chairman is a farmer. He sternly asserts, "Villagers should listen carefully to agricultural people." He wants Sister Hilary to back up his messages. The opening authoritative tone of the Headmaster seems to be reverberating in the Chairman's comments.

Sister Hilary probes. "Does the committee get support from the Chief and elders for their work?"

The Chairman responds. "Sister Hilary is a big person at the hospital, but sometimes she must holler at people to make them follow instructions." He has a complaint: "Each committee member has his own job. The Town Chief gives them absolutely no support." Everyone in the *barrie* claps. He clarifies, "The Section Chief does provide support. The committee wants to sit with the Chiefs so they can be given power. We can see that the Town Chief is absent. The Chief and elders knew you would be here tonight."

As though on cue, the Town Chief announces his arrival. In a show of support, the committee clerk indicates that the Town Chief has given him power to organize lodging and feeding of nurses. "This is now the responsibility of each different section head for the town."

The Town Chief nods, then utters not another word, sensing animosity towards him.

Sister asks, "If we stopped coming here for clinic, what would they do?"

The Chairman jumps in. "We'd ask why. We would beg you to continue coming."

Taking on a serious demeanour, Sister Hilary explains, "I would like them to know that the immunization is from the government. They have paid their hut taxes and should demand that we come."

Everyone claps approvingly.

Mama Hilary pursues another line of questioning. "Would they be interested in a health competition among section towns?"

Their reaction seems positive. "They need to discuss it further. Nobody will defeat them." Sister Hilary and I smile; Paul's forehead unfurls.

Paul prompts Sister Hilary to ask, "Why are their clinic numbers decreasing?"

The Section Chief explains. "At first, clinic numbers were good. Now there's a problem knowing when the nurses are coming, so we can't send out the town crier. The date for clinics should be set by the committee."

Sister Hilary nods and along the same lines suggests, "The committee should determine what they want to accomplish each year."

The committee Chairman responds quickly. "We've already decided to complete the maternity house. We are eager for new lessons and want to work strongly as a committee."

Sister Hilary's makes a parting remark in Krio: "*Let you take power for yourselves to go before.*"

Yengima

Sister Hilary begins: "You've had a village health committee for four years. What kinds of benefits have you seen here?"

The Chairman responds ardently: "We better understand sicknesses. People are no longer dying. We have clean drinking water in the dry season. People are using latrines; we are not seeing feces in the coffee plantation. The most important change is newborn tetanus; we no longer see it."

Sister Hilary praises the grannies who have encouraged women of child-bearing age to get their tetanus toxoid injections.

Another committee member continues, providing more examples of improvements. "We're not seeing difficulties associated with labour and delivery. We were not feeding our children properly. We now know what to feed *piken* to make them healthy and strong. We're no longer hand-feeding young babies. We're seeing less cough as a result. We now know the proper food for babies at three or four months, and we understand anemia."

Sister Hilary suggests that the committee members who responded should try for their nursing qualification. Committee members chuckle and nod vigorously. I think the student nurses who joined us tonight look a bit dejected; they are in the midst of studying for their national registration exams.

The man responsible for sanitation chimes in. "Most households have finished building their latrines. The first batch of cement was insufficient—they want more."

Sister Hilary responds, "We'll try to get you the cement we promised." She reminds them, "You can make latrines in the old way, with mud."

The Chairman brings up another point. "Some committee members were not attending meetings, so they made a few changes."

Sister Hilary replies, "I am pleased they made these changes themselves. The committee is for villagers. The fire must be from within."

They raise another problem. "We can't get nivaquine to treat malaria when the medicine man is away, and we can't afford to buy it."

Sister Hilary replies, "The few cents nivaquine costs isn't much for a life. The villagers need to try and pay for this medicine so Serabu Hospital can keep this medicine coming." There is no translated response to her remarks. Committee members' facial expressions suggest mixed opinions.

Paul and Simeon have floated the idea of a revolving fund for essential medicine. Our public health team needs to sort out the right structures for this kind of fund. It's hard to know how to introduce this notion. I think it's time to consult with market women and those with small shops to figure out how we can advance this idea.

Are We on the Right Path?

Taking-stock discussions were as vital to the village health work as home visits, clinics, and training for health committee members. I was intrigued by the back and forth that reinforced mutual account-abilities for public health work. The big bosses (Chiefs and Sister Hilary) raised and sorted challenges on both sides of the public health program equation. A stronger foundation was being forged between Serabu's public health team and villagers.

Cracks in the primary health care program were showing, driven by unsettling leadership dynamics in some communities, dodgy relationships between insiders and outsiders in a few places, and unrealistic expectations regarding people and material resources Serabu Hospital could provide.

Sister Hilary had reiterated the problem of TB. While Chiefs and village health committee members were willing to talk about *dry cough*, it had been at our behest. Chiefs had mentioned native healers who treated TB, but none of these healers had joined the meetings. A marked divide existed between Western and traditional approaches for treating *dry cough*.

Water and sanitation infrastructure improvements were inching along. Reports of more latrines in villages were small yet exciting achievements. Getting privies built required communal effort.

Follow-up was needed to determine if latrines were well-maintained and in common use, rather than being locked up except for visitors. We'd need to confirm that newly built wells met both technical requirements and cultural expectations; their location neither an insult nor a threat to the ancestors.

The under-belly of health work had been exposed. The balance between village dependence and independence teetered. What services and resources should communities expect of government? After all, families paid hut taxes. What free handouts was it reasonable for communities to expect from Serabu Hospital? The mission hospital had little government funding; this had been difficult to convey. What could the community provide? Feeding and lodging the nurses and offering free labour to build latrines and wells were common inputs. Village health committee members could avail themselves of the training offered by Serabu Hospital. They were keen to do so.

We heard stock answers when committee members explained their roles. We still needed to better understand how committee work aligned or interfered with occupations such as farming and seasonal mining.

Despite a sameness in village dialogues, challenges, successes, and social cohesion were unique to each community. Leadership support influenced committee members' pace of work. Gradual progress was being made. I was encouraged by village health committees' aspirations for better health.

The public health team's morale had been heisted, alongside a reality check. Change takes time. A few troubling, albeit unintended consequences, of Serabu's primary health care work had been reported. These needed attention. Where village health committees had been in place longer, community ownership was stronger. Yengima, one of the original three pilot villages, had described promising results. We were in a mutual learn-as-you-go experience.

We had heard what villagers considered health improvements. Health committees were no magic bullet, yet their members were motivated to continue. More training and reinforcement were needed. There was no straight line to better health.

Primary health care was hard work, not only for our public health team but also for committee members. Sometimes I took volunteer contributions of committee members for granted. They did health work *pan top* (on top of) the everyday struggle of their lives. This made their enthusiasm even more remarkable.

Extending village health committees to more communities was an overwhelming prospect. Discussions had sparked new ideas. Longer-standing health committees had a wealth of experience to share. Serabu's public health team needed to leverage this capacity without depleting the commitment and energy of committee members. Expansion was ripe with possibilities.

CHAPTER 16
DRY COUGH

Growing up, I heard family whispers about my paternal grandmother's sister, who died of TB in her teens. In high school, I learned that consumption had taken the lives of long-dead writers like Dickens and Bronte. My adolescent self, thought that TB was a disease of the past.

In university, nursing lectures had focused on TB in North America. The outlook was optimistic. The disease was in decline, sanatoriums had closed, and invasive surgical treatments for TB had ceased. TB screening was mandatory for health providers. By the 1970s, most TB patients in Canada received their drug therapy at home. TB remained a worrisome disease among the socially disadvantaged. It thrives in conditions of poverty. The prevalence of TB was highest among Canada's Indigenous populations.[20] Antibiotic resistance was concerning. Multi-drug treatment protocols were tackling that problem.

I got my annual Mantoux screening test and later a BCG vaccination when I went to work in Newfoundland. I had little direct clinical experience with TB patients. I knew the straight-forward basics of case finding and contact tracing.

TB in Sierra Leone

In Serabu, I found myself in the midst of a dismal TB problem. The disease was insidious. Menacing. Rife. When our public health team set out for village work, we had the names of TB patients referred to us by hospital staff. Some had not yet started their drug regimen. Others were taking oral medications after weeks of daily injections.

More had defaulted before completing their full course of treatment. All had contacts to trace. Serabu Hospital's public health nurses saw only the tip of the *dry cough* iceberg.

I imagined TB to be an underground vine, producing new cases along its runners while throwing up shoots of fear in its path. The penetrating vine adeptly grabbed the vulnerable: undernourished children, and adults with compromised health.

Villagers with symptoms of *dry cough* first consulted with traditional, not Western, health care providers. Traditional healers knew how to deal with the witches who were purveyors of *dry cough*. On this causal matter, the abilities of all Western care providers fell short.

Government Program

TB was not a new problem. For years, Serabu's physicians had tried to make headway. The government launched its TB control program in 1977. Serabu Hospital was an inaugural delivery site. The Sisters had guarded enthusiasm for the new initiative. It would bolster TB control efforts, although it offered no solutions to Serabu Hospital's workforce constraints.

The free government program included BCG immunizations, case finding, and treatment. The regimen for treating TB was long: a two- to three-month course of daily streptomycin injections followed by a year of oral medications. The control plan was straight-forward on paper, fraught in practice. It was typical of national TB plans of that era, riddled with assumptions about the super-structure of diagnostic, laboratory, and outreach services, and personnel available to roll it out. Plans read like they had been written by officials with their heads buried in urban sandpits.

In 1980, Sister Hilary wrote a memo on TB in Bumpe Chiefdom that had an uncharacteristically, pessimistic tone of defeat.[21] In that report, she described one patient in the Chiefdom who had received 33 visits by public health nurses. Despite the home visits, he had stopped taking his medication before completing his treatment regime.

Three years after the government program began, Serabu's physicians estimated an unwavering 3% TB prevalence rate in the villages of Bumpe Chiefdom.[22] No one knew how many active cases were in the Chiefdom. The hospital's register of TB patients provided a very incomplete picture of the problem; so few living with *dry cough* sought hospital treatment. Options for case finding were extremely limited.

Serabu Hospital had the only TB diagnostic equipment in Bumpe Chiefdom: a microscope for sputum tests and one X-ray machine that had been acquired ten years before my arrival. The single source of electricity in the Chiefdom was on the hospital compound. Procuring a portable X-ray machine for TB case finding was nonsensical. Sputum smear tests were done in Serabu Hospital's lab to confirm a diagnosis. Persuading a patient with a positive test to come for treatment was another matter, especially if symptoms were mild. For those who started but then prematurely stopped treatment, antibiotic resistance was a threat. The hospital pharmacy rarely stocked the more expensive second-line medications required to treat TB patients who developed drug resistance.

TB Control

Providing newly diagnosed TB patients with injections in their villages was unworkable. Serabu Hospital didn't have the manpower or transportation required to make this a viable option, not even in nearby villages. Some patients took up temporary housing near the hospital and came into the outpatient department for injections.

TB patients who stayed in Serabu must have fretted over unfulfilled child-care and household duties. Frailty prevented them from participating in vigorous farm work. Gaining strength must have fanned their guilt. Every person who didn't farm added to the potential food-per-person deficit.

Still, it was remarkable that nearly 80% of those who lodged in Serabu and started TB treatment stayed on for outpatient injections when they could have returned to their villages at any time.

Completing the streptomycin regimen was a major milestone. Finishing the phase of oral medications was another story.

TB patients determined they had been adequately treated when their symptoms abated. Stopping medications halted their side effects, bolstering patients' temporary sense of wellness. I assumed patients would view the switch from injections to oral medication to be a progressive transition in their treatment plan. Not so. Injections were considered to be more powerful medicine. Oral TB medications had to be taken for a full year, a sure indication of their dubious value. The lengthy period of therapy undermined patients' determination to beat the disease.

Lurking Witches

Dry cough was believed to be caused by a witch's spell. A *morie man* needed to be consulted to provide counter-measures: ceremonies, native herbs, and amulets. Only when these efforts failed did villagers come to the hospital to seek diagnosis and treatment. Most patients arrived with advanced TB.

Sister Hilary suggested one perceived advantage of coming to Serabu for treatment. By travelling a long distance, TB patients might "get out of range of local witches."[23] This same kind of thinking led some patients to leave one village for another, bringing the disease with them, expanding their network of contacts. These TB patients were literally on the run, seeking native medicine from traditional healers in other villages when their symptoms worsened. It wasn't hard to imagine that metaphorical witches were indeed perpetrating *dry cough*.

Patients' resolve to continue Western treatment diminished when they returned home. Serabu's physicians made no claims that their medicine provided protection from wrathful witches. Another consult was needed with a *morie man* to address the underlying and unresolved witch problem.

Our case-finding efforts may have reinforced beliefs in menacing witches. Questions about others with symptoms of active TB suggested that the witch danger lurked nearby.

TB patients lived on the fringes of their communities. Contact tracing meant disclosing their disease diagnosis to village leaders and to neighbours. *Dry cough* was steeped in stigma, increasing the risk of TB patients defaulting on medications and moving to other villages. The angst of those suffering from TB in remote villages must have verged on unbearable. These patients could be ostracized or *driven* from their communities.

Tiange lived in one of the three original primary health care villages. She was identified as a TB patient during annual physicals in Blama. She did not return for her annual physical in 1980. The Village Chief reported that she now lived in Mojajo. From Mojajo, she sought refuge in Mattine, where she got back on treatment. In each village, she had left a jumbled web of contacts behind.

Community Follow-up

Our public health team tried to locate and visit TB patients who had completed their first phase of treatment. These simple instructions involved complicated and resource-intensive logistics.

Kadiatu was a middle-aged mother, who had been discharged from the medical ward after completing her course of streptomycin injections. She was given a month's worth of oral medication to take home. Kadiatu needed to come back to the hospital for checkups and her supplies of isoniazid and thiazine. We were asked to assess her progress and do contact tracing.

I had the name of her village. I stood squinting in front of the large, detailed map of Bumpe Chiefdom that was tacked onto the tutor's office wall. I searched the tiny print for the village name and exclaimed when I found it. Then I found a second and a third village with the same name. My enthusiasm drained. Reaching these villages involved setting out in different directions from the hospital, traversing bush-paths and swamps.

Our public health team took a guess and headed off, hoping we'd selected the correct village. We weren't lucky; we didn't find the patient until we set out a third time. We located a few of her household members and inquired of TB symptoms. Any cough, weight loss, or blood in their sputum? I was skeptical about their answers. Who would divulge their symptoms when they knew we had come to see someone with TB? We obtained sputum samples, hoping suspect cases had coughed deeply enough to provide test-worthy phlegm.

Kadiatu had said she would come to Serabu's outpatient clinic every month to collect her oral medication. I figured her return visits were highly improbable.

Plodding On

TB remained pervasive and malicious. Case finding and follow-up meant more village treks, better detective work to locate contacts, and stronger health messages to reinforce the need for lengthy Western treatment. Serabu's public health efforts paled in comparison with the hardships shouldered by TB patients and their families. We reassured ourselves that our community efforts slowed the spread of TB. We brought willing Chiefs and village health committee members on board as hospital-staff extenders. They observed the ingestion of TB drugs by patients in their villages, encouraging them to finish treatment. We urged communities to support rather than shun *dry cough* patients.

Some patients had completed TB treatment. New patients had been diagnosed after contact tracing. Yet, it was hard not to be cynical. The odds were against us. Breaking through *dry cough's* tenacious stigma was near impossible. Even if we had thrown all of Serabu's public health resources at case finding and treatment, I was unconvinced we'd make a substantial dent in the problem. BCG immunizations promised the best long-term results. We upped those efforts.

Our public health team plodded on with glimmers of hope. Possibly, TB-control efforts eroded stigma, pressed patients with active TB to seek treatment earlier, and encouraged those who were on the last leg of their treatment protocol to finish. No formulaic path could resolve this obstinate problem. *Dry cough* was arrogant and predatory; a trickster better equipped to gain the upper hand than Serabu's physicians and nurses. Dealing the disease a death blow was impossible.

CHAPTER 17
TRADITIONAL BIRTH ATTENDANTS

Post-independence, Sierra Leone's government had strengthened maternal and child health services for the country's rural areas by training auxiliary workers. Village maternity assistants were the first trainees, followed by better-prepared MCH aides.

By the mid-1970s, it was apparent that deploying auxiliary workers had not brought about the desired improvements in neonatal, infant, or maternal mortality rates. TBAs were still attending the majority of births: 70% of all births in Sierra Leone, and 85% of all deliveries in Bumpe Chiefdom.

Dr. Belmont Williams, the Chief Medical Officer (CMO) took a bold decision. In 1974, she established government training for TBAs to improve maternal and neonatal care in rural areas. This three-week course was offered at several provincial and district hospitals once or twice a year, with an enrolment of 30 or so in each training cohort.[24] By the time I arrived in Serabu, several hundred TBAs from across Sierra Leone had received government training, including a handful from Bumpe Chiefdom.

How TBAs Described Their Work

The roles of TBAs were rooted in Mende culture and in the women's Secret Society. TBAs' beliefs, practices, and community identities were interwoven. They had earned intergenerational respect for their prowess as midwives. Many had a proven track record delivering healthy babies. They were revered for their dual roles as birth attendants and as members or leaders of the *Bundu* Society. TBAs were the preferred provider.

TBAs were keen to explain their work, inviting me, along with other female members of our public health team, into delivery huts in the *Bundu* bush. This is where they disclosed *women's business*.

I asked TBAs how they were selected. Two responses were common. Most were chosen by a practising TBA to become an apprentice due to their lineage (having an Auntie or other relative who was a TBA). Apprenticeship was not a set length. From the beginning, birth attendants assisted with labour and delivery. As the health of an established granny midwife failed, assistant TBA(s) took over the lead role. Other TBAs described a self-selection process. Some had unexpectedly attended a delivery. *Ngewo* had guided them. Others had dreamt of doing a delivery and then taken on this work.

Deliveries were usually conducted by groups of TBAs: the head and her assistants, each of them guiding the others, as a woman progressed through labour and delivery. The work of TBAs did not stop with a delivery. During the post-partum period, they supported women to breastfeed and rest; dressed infants' umbilical cords; brought infants out into daylight on their third or fourth day of life (a practice directly translated as presenting the infant to the street); and participated in naming ceremonies.

I was invited to witness the naming ceremony for baby Bendu. It was an intimate village celebration of life. Bendu slept through the entire affair.

Journal Entry

September 24th, 1980

Blama

Three metal pans are placed in front of mother and baby. Two contain pounded rice with honey and kola nuts on top; the third pan holds Le 3 worth of coins. Kola brings good luck to parents and child, honey is for good health always, and money is given in lieu of expensive items such as salt. A long Muslim prayer is recited by all—arms extended, hands pointing towards the offerings. Bendu has been blessed. The community has wrapped its arms around the newborn as she starts life's journey.

Serabu Hospital's TBA Training and Supervision

Although many TBAs had firsthand experience attending complicated deliveries, Serabu Hospital was the delivery location recommended for high-risk pregnant women. With training, normal deliveries in the villages would be safer, and granny midwives would know who to send to hospital. Sister Hilary considered TBA upskilling to be a vital part of the primary health care program. She wrote a letter to TBAs conveying her regard for their work, and inviting them to participate in training. The invitation was issued via Village Chiefs.

An Invitation for TBAs to Join Serabu Hospital's Training Program[25]

To the Midwife:

You live in a village that is far from a hospital, a nurse, or a doctor. For hundreds of years, you and your ancestors have taken care of the arrival of children into this world.

You have found out many things about causes and treatments. You have done well. You have kept the tribe alive and multiplying. Since you were young, many new things and new sense have come in the world. We bring some of these to you to help you better.

We would like to put our two heads together—the old and the new, so that child bearing may be even safer than before.

The most important thing for you to know is that all normal cases are delivered in their home, and only the difficult ones go to the hospital.

We would like you to share with us the knowledge of the old times so we do not forget. We will share ours with you.

Villages with health committees were a priority for TBA training. The aim was to reduce maternal and neonatal morbidity and mortality rates. Sister Hilary developed a curriculum with ten lessons. The content was similar to that of government TBA training with the exception of family planning. That subject was not part of Serabu's curriculum.

Lessons addressed the common problems that TBAs dealt with in their work. Pregnancy topics included antenatal clinic, nutrition, and danger signs like bleeding and anemia. Content about deliveries covered preparation for a normal delivery, when to refer a *belly woman* (pregnant woman) to hospital, resuscitating newborns, and preventing newborn tetanus. A third set of lessons concerned the postpartum period: care of the mother and baby after delivery, complications requiring hospital referral, and registering births and deaths.

All TBAs resident in a village were invited to participate in training sessions, even those who were too old to conduct deliveries. This was consistent with their usual group practice for deliveries.

Serabu's lead TBA trainer was Sister Denise. Marcella provided cultural and language translation. Teaching took place in *Bundu* huts, giving trainers a firsthand look at TBAs' work conditions and equipment. Grannies were eager for lessons.

TBAs adapted lesson content to Mende tunes. They sang the lyrics time and again. TBAs re-enacted deliveries through role-playing. New procedures for existing equipment were introduced, like sterilizing the bamboo sliver or razor blade used to cut a baby's cord. A homemade doll, complete with umbilical cord and placenta, was used for demonstration purposes.

Grannies who were too frail to walk to another village could take part. Older TBAs were influential, especially those who held leadership positions in the *Bundu* Society. They coached younger and less experienced midwives and could persuade other TBAs to adopt new practices.

Journal Entry

October 24th, 1980

Blama

I'm surprised to see four TBAs in such a small village. One old and clever granny is no longer hands-on for deliveries because her eyesight has deteriorated. Her spirit and enthusiasm for the work are still strong; she is anxious to show us that she does remember lessons taught to her about high-risk pregnancies.

The head midwife, Isatu, cannot recollect how many deliveries she has done. She takes off her white head tie to show us her grey hairs in response to our questions about her age and experiences. The other TBAs tell us that Isatu has delivered four generations of mothers. Isatu has two assistants, both are young mothers with *strong hearts* [courage]; she is anxious for them to attend lessons. They want a nurse to come to the village to teach them every two weeks. They would like to learn by watching deliveries in the hospital.

TBA training piqued curiosity. Other village women asked to listen in. A subtle shift in pregnant women's expectations of TBAs began.

Sister Denise tried out numerous training schedules, settling on a couple of hours, one morning a week, before TBAs went to their farms. On average, it took 12 to 20 sessions to complete all lessons. Training was time- and transport-intensive.

Once grannies demonstrated their understanding of lessons, the trainer held an oral and practical examination. TBAs were invited to role-play how they conducted a normal delivery. They assembled their equipment for a delivery: a clean straw mat and *lappa;* a kettle for boiling the string and blade; a new razor blade, soap, and a wash basin; and *omolie* to clean the umbilical cord. Questions tested their knowledge. Who should be referred to hospital for delivery? How can *soin-soin* be prevented? Why tell a *belly woman* to attend antenatal clinic? Most TBAs passed the test. They were well practised in advance of this formality.

I wondered about grannies who did not pass. Were they humiliated or intimidated? Did the test motivate them to continue learning or did failure leave them discouraged? I had the impression that those who succeeded encouraged other TBAs to take more lessons until they earned their certificate. Their long-standing cultural practices were collegial. TBAs were not pitted one against another for a position on the delivery team.

Certificate ceremonies were a big deal. The majority of TBAs had no formal schooling. Their training-completion certificate was the first they had ever held in their hands, never mind earned for themselves. They beamed with pride during award ceremonies, as other villagers and the Chief or his Speaker gathered in the village *barrie* to recognize their achievement. Sister Hilary attended as the hospital dignitary.

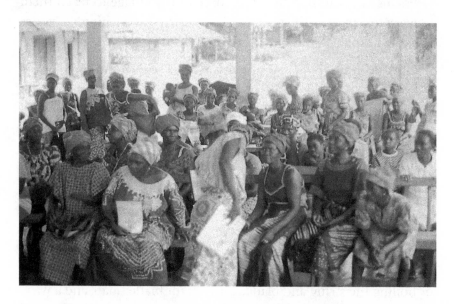

TBAs gathered in a barrie to receive Serabu Hospital training certificates
(Bumpe Chiefdom).

Awarding certificates was a public way of stating that TBAs were expected to implement what they had learned. It reinforced their accountability for safe deliveries to the community. There was a place on the certificate to write the date of re-examination. Gently, but firmly, Sister Hilary explained that a certificate could be withdrawn if a granny was found negligent in her practice.

Our public health team encouraged trained TBAs to participate in antenatal clinics. With supportive supervision, they improved their abilities to get a clinical history; palpate the abdomen; check for anemia, edema, and other risk factors; and explain the importance of tetanus toxoid immunization. Involving TBAs in village clinics reinforced our message that they were part of a larger health care team. We hoped this would encourage high-risk pregnant women to come to hospital for delivery.

Each rendezvous with granny midwives was an eye-opener for me. I admired their genuine comradery and the solidarity of their woman-power. I loved their enthusiasm for midwifery work.

Journal Entries

October 25th, 1980

Bangor

As soon as the traditional midwife sees us, she goes into her room to get a frayed cloth bag. She pulls out a book for registering births. She is illiterate. Each birth has been entered with someone's assistance. The last recorded birth is October 23rd, 1980, two days ago. Given all the entries, she must do a thriving business.

The TBAs lead us to a round hut. Posters advertising Guinness and Geritol are pasted on the mud wall, alongside a tattered and faded picture of Dustin Hoffman. A mob of school-age children gather round and peer in through the open shutters. They are sent running with shouts from the granny midwives who announce that we're going to talk *women's business*. The maternity assistant, who was trained in Serabu, is in attendance. She is not an active midwife because of a drinking problem.

Social Disruption

Sometimes, well-intentioned training was a source of social disruption. I heard an example of this during a visit to Sahn, where a government-trained TBA had been deployed to the village without the knowledge or input of resident TBAs. This was an affront, creating unwanted competition for deliveries.

Journal Entry

October 27th, 1980

Sahn

> Sahn's TBAs take us to their *Bundu* house. The hospital midwife, a nursing student, and I are invited to sit with the TBAs on two old wood cots in the stuffy, mud-walled room. We squeeze into narrow spaces between the seated TBAs, hips and thighs touching, our bums sinking into the concave straw mattresses. There are eight grannies in Sahn. They explain that families of pregnant women select the TBA or TBAs they want to do the delivery. Even when only one granny is chosen, several traditional midwives are in attendance.

> The TBAs have a quandary. At the request of their Section and Village Chiefs, the Paramount Chief sent a government-trained TBA to their village to do deliveries. The request bypassed these grannies. They claim they don't even know the name of this trained TBA. They are upset because she is taking away their business. She charges Le 8 to deliver a boy and Le 6 for a girl. I'm surprised at the prices; a hospital delivery in Serabu costs Le 6. The midwives are doubly upset because even if they go to help the recently trained TBA, they're not given anything, no remuneration. They are under the erroneous impression that the trained TBA goes to Bo to collect a salary.

> I wondered if those in charge of the government TBA training were aware of this unfortunate situation.

A Maternal Death

TBA training was not without its problems, but our public health team was encouraged by the rising demand for TBA training and early results. Approximately 18 months after TBAs and other village health committee members had been trained in 11 villages and towns, we conducted a follow-up survey. The neonatal tetanus and infant mortality rates were dropping. We attributed this to the combined impact of village health committees, TBA training, and immunizations. Although we were on the right track, we had a long ways to go. We had reached only a small portion of villages in Bumpe Chiefdom, and the maternal death rate remained stubbornly high.

Around that time, a jarring event occurred. Word reached Sister Hilary about a tragic incident involving a young pregnant teenager. After agonizing hours in obstructed labour, this youngster died in a deplorable and unnecessary way. The grannies who attended her were not trained. If the teen had been referred to Serabu Hospital, a caesarian section would have saved her life and maybe her newborn's.

I had never seen Sister Hilary so distraught. She set out to the village immediately after hearing the news. She was barely keeping a lid on her outrage, and expounded on the unacceptable circumstances of the teen's demise. In no uncertain terms she told the village leaders "This must never, ever happen again."

Sista Docta Hilary handed the matter over to the Chiefs and the health committee of the nearby section town. They were instructed to come back to Serabu Hospital with a solution. Two weeks later, the community health department received a message requesting that we send a nurse to teach the TBAs involved in the incident how to do a better job. They were to join monthly training sessions along with other TBAs from the same section of villages. Twenty-five TBAs signed on for and attended classes.

TBA Training Bottleneck

Our public health team wanted to reach more TBAs and more villages, but we had run into a significant bottleneck. Bumpe Chiefdom had 236 villages. We had no register of TBAs; their exact numbers were unknown. Even in smaller villages, three or four TBAs practised midwifery. Serabu had nine TBAs. We estimated there were hundreds of untrained traditional midwives in Bumpe Chiefdom.

Sister Denise had other work responsibilities on the maternity ward. If we persisted with the strategy of one nurse-midwife doing all the training and maintained our peak rate of training TBAs in 12 to 13 villages a year, we estimated it would take two decades to train all TBAs in the Chiefdom.

Trained TBAs had to be supervised. They would need refresher lessons. New TBAs would begin midwifery work. Our discouraging estimates of the coverage rate were overly optimistic.

MCH aides were an alternative resource for TBA training. With four aides in Bumpe Chiefdom, the MCH aide per population ratio was approximately 1:8,000—reasonably close to the 1:6,000 ratio targeted by the Ministry of Development. Engaging MCH aides as trainers was consistent with the lines of referral TBAs were taught to follow; village to health centre to hospital.

If MCH aides were to be effective TBA trainers and supervisors, two important sources of conflict needed to be dealt with: prestige and money. The root of these problems was that MCH aides started off as strangers in the communities where they were deployed. Government posted them to villages where they were needed. An MCH aide was in direct competition with TBAs for births. Every delivery a TBA did was Le 10 an MCH aide did not earn, while every delivery an MCH aide did was payment in kind or cash that granny midwives did not collect. MCH aides got a stipend from the government, but it was inadequate. They had to supplement their government income to get by.

MCH aides had not been trained for 18 months to do the job of a TBA. Rather they were the first referral point for granny midwives and could pass on knowledge and skills to improve TBAs' work. Sister Hilary and Sister Denise reckoned that MCH aides should be more involved in TBA training.

CHAPTER 18
BREAKDOWNS AND BREAKTHROUGHS

Serabu Hospital staff depended on TBAs to initiate referrals of pregnant, labouring, and postpartum women from the villages. Obstetrical emergencies like bleeding, obstructed labour, and breech presentations were major concerns. Initiating a referral was one thing, orchestrating a timely referral to a hospital was quite another. There were delays in seeking care, reaching care, and receiving care.[26] Systemic referral barriers were formidable.

The husband or uncle of a woman was the family member who had the cultural authority to give permission for a woman to be admitted to hospital. This was a social safeguard. Among poor farmers, whose households earned, on average, less than Le 12 per month, a decision to send a woman to hospital involved pooling scarce resources to cover costs. This cash outlay meant foregoing other essentials like school fees or transport to take produce to market. Sending someone to hospital could jettison an extended family into debt.

If a pregnant woman was identified as high risk, pre-emptive decisions about paying for the cost of a hospital delivery could take place. However, untrained TBAs were unfamiliar with the notion of high-risk status. If male family heads needed to confer about payment for transport and hospital fees when an obstetrical emergency arose, this often delayed referrals by hours or days. When household heads were unreachable, a hospital-admission decision was unresolvable.

Accessible transportation was lacking. Even when a woman lived in a so-called motorable village, it was near impossible to hire a vehicle to transport a patient experiencing an obstetrical emergency. During the day, roadworthy private vehicles were in nearly-constant use and packed with paying customers. No driver wanted to disrupt regular business to carry a seriously ill patient to hospital. Furthermore, desperate villagers had no way to contact drivers while they were on their routes. At night, when vehicles were parked, families might beg a driver to use his vehicle as an ambulance. Since drivers were rarely owners of their vehicles, they were unable to authorize this alternative use.

Poda-poda owners were reticent to have their vehicles deployed as pseudo-ambulances. They did not want to be held responsible for a possible maternal death, a hemorrhaging pregnant or postpartum woman, or a newborn delivery gone awry en route to hospital.

Serabu Hospital didn't have an ambulance, although we occasionally transported patients in the utility van. I recall a critically ill pregnant woman who was brought to the village where we were holding an evening immunization clinic. She was unconscious and convulsing relentlessly due to eclampsia. Her family had agreed she should be taken to hospital. Two wiry men had carried her in a hammock strung through a bamboo pole that rested on their shoulders. We laid the patient on the metal floor of the van, tucking a couple of *lappas* under her to provide some miniscule semblance of cushioning for the bumpy drive. We had no medications with us to treat her condition. The driver sped back to Serabu as Simeon and I crouched beside the moribund patient, willing her to hold on. She survived; her infant was stillborn.

A postpartum hemorrhage was one of the most feared childbirth complications because there was so little time to act. Many TBAs had seen or heard of women bleeding heavily after childbirth, sometimes with lethal consequences. When mothers died during or after childbirth, their infants almost never survived.

Massaging the fundus of the uterus after birth reduced excessive bleeding. Nurses taught TBAs how to do this. However, when a hemorrhage occurs, the main intervention required is an injection of ergometrine that contracts the uterus and stops bleeding. This life-saving drug was inconsistently stocked in peripheral health units.

The impossibility of getting a hemorrhaging postpartum woman to a hospital in time to save her life crystallized for me when I visited Komende, a village on the other side of the Jong River. I had travelled there with students to conduct a community needs assessment. On the map, and as the crow flies, the destination village was just a few miles from a mission hospital run by the Methodists in Mattru-Jong. Our trip to that village relayed a different geographic narrative.

It took us half a day and three modes of transportation to get there. We began with a 20-minute vehicle ride from the hospital to a village by the river. We then walked alongside three miles of rice paddies. We needed to get across the river. Florence was the lightweight student in our group. Without hesitation, she climbed a tree and hollered for a boatman to give us a ride in his slim dugout canoe. Safely on the other side, we walked another mile through local farms to reach our destination. This was the harsh reality: A woman with a postpartum hemorrhage in Komende would bleed out before she got to the "local" hospital. In the darkness of night, the route was impassible.

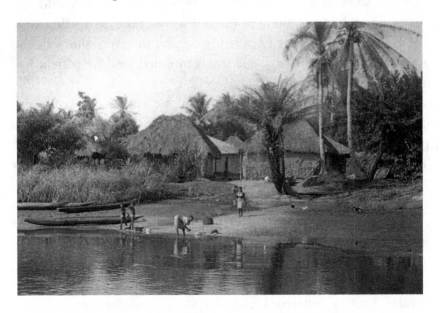

En route to Komende, a village on Jong River (Mattru-Jong Chiefdom).

A plethora of circumstances thwarted timely referrals; each added delays. From my perspective, the bottlenecks looked almost insurmountable. From the perspective of a woman and her family, barriers must have seemed cataclysmic.

A Referral System Gone Awry

The hospital's lights were still on even though it was past the blackout hour. Anne and I had heard a commotion coming from outside the maternity ward where a lorry had driven up. Shortly after, we saw Sister Sheila, Serabu's lead surgeon, stride to the operating theatre for the urgent obstetrical case.

News of this patient spread quickly among staff the next morning. She had arrived in obstructed labour; her condition was grim. Her circuitous journey had started in the Eastern Province, which was well outside the geographic catchment area for Serabu Hospital. She had been sent from her village to the provincial hospital in Kenema, and then 44 miles to Bo's provincial hospital. At both government facilities, she and her accompanying family member were told that the personnel and equipment needed for a caesarian section were not available. The woman arrived in Serabu in severe shock due to a ruptured uterus. Sister Sheila was astounded that the patient had survived the harrowing journey.

Given broken chains in the referral system, the horrific outcomes that unfolded for this woman were inevitable. Sister Sheila performed a life-saving hysterectomy. Her baby was macerated. The young woman lived but she could no longer bear children. Her social situation had changed immeasurably.

Along with other staff, I lamented this tragic case for days. I had emotional and emotive discussions about this patient at home and in the classroom. The young woman's losses were utterly preventable. There was no making sense of this particular situation; no coming to terms with it. I was stupefied by the impossibility of such a desperately broken obstetrical referral system. Cynicism cast a shadow in my mind. Many more women in the villages had suffered the dire consequences of obstetrical emergencies, having never made it to a health facility. The immensity of the problem made me weep.

The referral chain for maternity patients was completely broken. Chaotically dysfunctional. Beyond repair. Provincial government hospitals were increasingly ill-equipped to deal with emergencies. Their medical supplies and basic drugs were running short. Operating theatres were out of commission during lengthy electrical blackouts. Essentials, like sterilized equipment, were intermittently available. Barely a handful of physicians were on staff. Although registered midwives managed some difficult deliveries, physicians were required for caesarian sections.

With time, my heaviness lifted. I found reasons to be optimistic again. In the midst of the tragedy were successes. High-risk women had made it to Serabu Hospital in time for caesarian sections or forceps' deliveries. Serabu's maternity ward was full of higher-risk mothers breastfeeding their healthy newborns. Lower-risk pregnant women had been safely delivered by TBAs.

Communication Breakdowns

TBAs were lynch pins for referrals. With training, they could identify signs of trouble during pregnancy like anemia, vaginal bleeding, swollen feet, lethargy, and persistent headaches. They were the first to suspect that a woman's labour was not progressing normally. TBAs encouraged household heads to consider the unthinkable— sending a wife or relative to hospital for delivery rather than birthing in the community. Granny midwives provided the crucial liaison between villages and hospital. However, there had to be a receptive health provider at the hospital if a seamless referral was to take place.

By the time registered nurse-midwives and physicians graduated, they had been taught repeatedly that high-risk pregnant women, if not all women in labour, should be brought to a hospital for delivery and without delay. This thinking shaped their attitudes and demeanour. Serious communication breakdowns occurred when trained health professionals gave referral instructions to pregnant women or TBAs that did not align with village realities. Referrals were threatened by unfortunate interactions that sometimes took place between TBAs and hospital personnel, pitching birth attendant training efforts backwards.

A trained TBA, resident in a village not too far from Bo's government hospital, gave a vivid account of such interactions gone awry. Speaking in Krio, she shared her tumultuous experience with me. She had vowed never to go back to Bo's maternity ward following an incident with hospital staff.

She had brought a woman, who had been in labour for two days, to the government hospital for admission. This TBA had spent long hours attending the woman and a sleepless night persuading the patient's husband to let his wife go to hospital. He had relented on one condition: the traditional midwife, the provider he trusted, had to stay with his wife throughout her hospitalization.

The charge nurse and staff midwife had shown the TBA a total lack of respect when she arrived with the labouring woman at the hospital entrance. They shouted at her, asking why she had waited so long. They had not even given her a chance to explain the legitimate reason for the delay. Instead, the nurse and midwife made disparaging remarks and banished her from the hospital and from the patient who was in her care. This granny midwife had been forced to break her promise to the woman and her husband. The confrontation threatened to fracture her relationship with her community. When she spoke to me, she was still feeling wretched about the whole affair.

Her story shocked my sensibilities. What was the point of training TBAs if hospital-based health professionals were not on side? I knew there was a lot to be desired about the clinical practices of TBAs, but on this matter I fully supported the granny midwife. Referring high-risk women to hospital was critical; TBAs knew this was way more complex than simply telling a woman to seek hospital care. TBA training needed to bridge this divide between traditional TBAs and Western-trained practitioners.

Granny midwives were implicated in any referral improvements we conjured up. Respectful communication between traditional and

Western-trained health providers was the foundation for a functional system.

The TBA emboldened me to drive a new message home. I have used her powerful anecdote over and over again in national and international meetings. I extend her a long overdue thanks for sharing her intimate and insightful story with me. It touched and taught me deeply.

A Cultural Breakthrough

Alongside referral bottlenecks that kept maternal mortality rates high were situations that gave me hope. One of these is seared in my optimistic memory bank because it signalled a pivotal change that would save the lives of many newborns.

When I first arrived in Serabu, I was astounded by the prevalence of neonatal tetanus. Sierra Leone was on the World Health Organization's dismal, top-ten list for this disease. In rural areas of Sierra Leone, one quarter of all infant deaths were due to this disease. How was this possible? For me, the risk of tetanus brought to mind dirty-nail puncture wounds, necessitating a doctor's appointment to make sure tetanus toxoid immunization was up to date. I was a tetanus neophyte. I'd never seen a patient with tetanus. I vaguely knew that what the locals called *soin-soin,* was a thing.

The horrible truth had sunk in. Tetanus took the lives of many newborns in Bumpe Chiefdom. All health providers agreed that this unabated suffering of babies and mothers had to stop.

Neonatal tetanus was common for a number of reasons. Most pregnant women and their newborns had no immunity to this disease. Mass tetanus toxoid immunization was not introduced until 1978. This was a vaccine access, not an anti-vax issue.

Newborns were infected through their umbilical cords. Typically, granny midwives did not wash their hands before a delivery. Women normally delivered their babies while lying on the earthen floor of the *Bundu* hut. Cord-cutting tools were commonly stored, unwrapped, in the mud-wall cracks of delivery huts and neither washed nor sterilized before use. To aid cord healing, some TBAs covered the umbilical stump with native medicine, which they innocently mixed with dirt, clay, or charcoal. These practices created perfect conditions for tetanus spores to enter a baby's cord stump and wreak neurotoxic havoc.

Every mother and every granny midwife feared *soin-soin*. No ifs, ands, or buts. Without treatment, a newborn with tetanus would die. We knew it, TBAs knew it, and mothers knew it. Even with in-hospital treatment, a baby's chance of surviving tetanus was slim. Most infants who developed *soin-soin* went untreated. The disease kills cruelly and swiftly. Few cases made it to hospital. Besides, treatment was no answer for this completely preventable baby killer.

Serabu's public health team was united in its determination to stamp out this disease. A *marcleate* for a pregnant woman prevented tetanus for her newborn. With each and every clinic, village assessment, TBA training session, antenatal home visit, and discussion with a local Chief, we emphasized the necessity of tetanus toxoid immunization for all women of child-bearing age. Immunization rates began to climb. Community assessments confirmed a subsequent drop in neonatal tetanus cases. Nevertheless, immunization rates remained low in many villages. Prevention messaging was still being driven by Serabu's public health team and hospital staff, rather than by Mende women and TBAs.

A quiet undercurrent of change bloomed one momentous day. I was teaching in the classroom. The louvered windows were open to let the morning breeze waft over us. Mid-lesson, the students and I were distracted by singing. Then our full attention was drawn by a *Sowei* leading a group of *Bundu* Society initiates. They danced in unison from outside the maternity ward as they headed towards the public health office. The teens wore long strings of beads draped around their necks and colourful *lappas* tied around their waists.

Sister Hilary joined us. The *Sowei* stepped forward and enthusiastically explained why they had come. Unbeknownst to us, the local TBAs had decided that tetanus toxoid immunizations should become part of their initiation rituals.

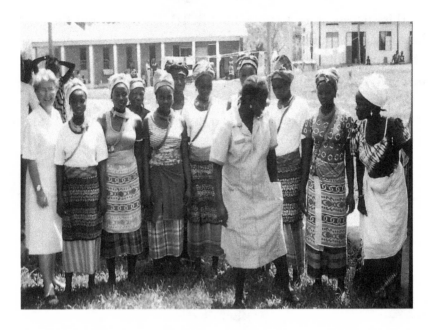

New Bundu Society initiates with Sowei (right), Sister Hilary (left), and Marcella Reffell speaking to Sowei. Surgical and maternity wards of Serabu Hospital in background.

Sister Hilary responded with affection, on behalf of the public health team. "We would be honoured to bring the tetanus toxoid immunizations to the initiates in the *Bundu* bush."

Our beaming faces conveyed our hearty endorsement of the TBAs' decision. I was over the moon with excitement. I put a pause on the classroom lesson that now seemed trivial. We joined the *Sowei* and initiates in their soft-shuffle dancing.

The *Sowei's* pronouncement was a major turning point. *Bundu* Society leaders had signalled that the solution to *soin-soin* was now owned by the Mende women themselves. Tetanus preventive practices had been re-envisioned and culturally integrated. There was no going back. At the invitation of the TBAs, we had joined forces as pro-vaxers. Together, we'd stamp out the dreaded *soin-soin*. There would be fewer baby boys named *Jibao* and baby girls named *Lumbeh*—Mende names meaning let this one live.

This success story left me, the SECHN students, and the public health team exhilarated. The TBAs were already spreading word of this new initiation practice among their *sister* granny midwives in other villages. Henceforth, initiates in Bumpe Chiefdom could expect female members of Serabu's public health team to join them in the *Bundu* bush to administer two complimentary rounds of tetanus toxoid immunizations.

PART 4
LEAVING AND RETURNING TO SIERRA LEONE
1981-1984

"The moon stays bright when it doesn't avoid the night." (Rumi)

CHAPTER 19
A PIVOT POINT

Around my fourth month in the country, I extended my CUSO contract for a third year in Serabu when it became crystal clear that I had much to learn before I could make any substantial contributions. I had committed to a 12-month extension without hesitation. As I contemplated whether and how to spend a fourth year in the country, questions about my future career directions were starting to erupt. Long-term work in international development was an appealing route—but with what organization, in which countries, and in what capacity?

I had questioned whether short-term efforts contributed to a sustainable development process. I had seen reinforcing, incremental wins and perceptible shifts in mindsets, practices, and expectations. Ultimately, the drivers of change were community members themselves. I was confident that some of the positive changes I had witnessed in Bumpe Chiefdom would be self-sustaining. I felt more rooted in Mende culture. I was proud of the nursing students' accomplishments.

Still, I was unsettled. Sierra Leone was my temporary home. I was looking forward to being closer to family. I was conscious of my ticking biological clock. I hoped to marry and have children. The prospects for same lay in Canada, not in Sierra Leone.

I had applied to graduate school. My application was accepted. A stint in the Design, Measurement, and Evaluation master's program at McMaster University would give me time to sort out future directions. I applied for a fellowship from the Canadian International Development Agency (CIDA). The application required a description of graduate studies and research in a third-world country.

Research had to be conducted either as part of, or immediately after, completing graduate degree requirements. I chose the latter. I put forward a plan that would bring me back to Sierra Leone to undertake the research project that I would design to meet thesis completion requirements.

I described my research topic as the selection, preparation, and ongoing training of village health workers and the cost-effectiveness of training and participatory evaluation of illiterate village health workers. While I contemplated an exclusive focus on TBAs, this idea was in my head rather than in my application. I was a long ways from having an adequately focused research question.

If I received the fellowship, coming back to Sierra Leone for a year would be a good place to consolidate my soon-to-be-acquired research skills. My fellowship application was successful. My departure was going to be temporary. I felt relieved.

Reconnecting with Family

I spent time with my parents and siblings in Vancouver before and after my year of graduate studies. Although I had sent them regular correspondence from Sierra Leone, my family had pent-up questions. I had written frequently, usually on standard one-and-a-half page aerogrammes. When international guests offered to post letters from abroad, I'd hastily scribble notes so as not to miss the services of self-appointed couriers. There were big gaps in what I divulged.

My early letters were full of initial impressions: the hospital compound and the small house where I lived; my students and co-workers, work schedules, and transportation to villages; and how friendly people were. I had lots to say about the food we were eating, tropical vegetation, amenities in Bo, and my struggles learning Mende.

In contrast, my descriptions of the public health work were cryptic. "Last week we held mass immunizations in ten different villages and immunized nearly 2,000 children. I feel like I've heard every child in Sierra Leone cry."

My younger sister, Sheila, who is a nurse, got a few more details about the medical conditions I was seeing, in my letters to her. "The children's ward is like an intensive care unit … We are finding loads of open TB cases and there are marasmic children … Last week [we found] a child unconscious with meningitis. All the villagers were gathered around him when we unexpectedly arrived."

My correspondence took on a distinctive pattern. I started with quick updates; my work responsibilities; the comings and goings of international visitors. I conveyed more complete descriptions of Irish Sisters and volunteers, than of Sierra Leonean students and colleagues. My mother is of Irish stock. I figured stories about the Irish Sisters and volunteers provided an inroad for my family to relate to my Serabu experiences.

When hungry season encroached, I opted for factual content. "This is the hungry time of the year; very little rice is available. Children seem to suffer the most. We are seeing more malnutrition." I did not disclose how overwhelmed the disease burden and suffering made me feel.

I shared my excitement at the prospect of using a local loom. My family sent me a textile-weaving book. I let them know when I had planted cotton seeds, and when shoots popped up. That multi-letter tale culminated with my report of an agricultural failure: "I picked cotton off my one surviving plant today—barely enough to spin a ten-inch thread."

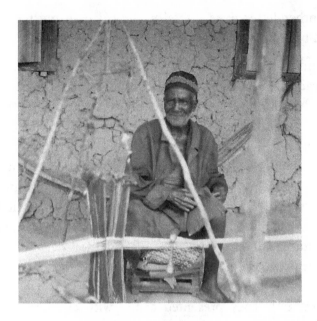

Country-cloth weaver using traditional loom. Country cloth was woven in six- to eight-inch wide strips using locally spun cotton thread. Imported black thread was sometimes used for the long narrow stripe patterns. Cloth strips were sewn together to make blankets.

I did not intend to write letters with shock-value, but that is how some of my stories were experienced.

Last Monday, I went to Mattru with 27 students [for community assessments] ... I travelled around the Chiefdom and visited all of the students, making sure there were no problems. Female students met with TBAs to teach them skills like careful handwashing and boiling the razor blade and string before cutting and tying the cord. Some of the information students gathered is amazing. One woman who reported that 11 of her 12 children had died of tetanus, lives in the village of Mattru, where there is a hospital. Another woman had given birth to eight; all had died of newborn tetanus.

In another letter, I described a clinical case my family found downright perplexing.

> Sudima's story will give you some insight into the traditional beliefs that so strongly influence people's behaviour. One of my students translated what the baby's father said. Sudima, age five months, is from Lugbo Chiefdom. Her mother is the only wife of her husband. She has given birth to seven children. Just two are alive. The fifth child died of headache and fever. The other children were believed to have died of witchcraft. The parents are farmers. They blamed Sudima's illness on witchcraft, so they decided to perform ceremonies by sacrificing a cock by the riverside at night to beg the witches [to not harm Sudima]. They presented a hen with clean rice to the biggest cotton tree in their village as an apology for the wrongdoing [of the witches] to their other children. They performed the ceremonies and gave much native medicine to Sudima but there was still no improvement in the child's condition.

How puzzling this raw anecdote must have been for my family. I provided no description of Sudima's diagnosis or hospital treatment, and no statement regarding her prognosis. My description of witchcraft left my family baffled. I communicated no hint of my own bewilderment and disquiet about the family's ceremonies.

Worry Suppressant Techniques

My father was an engineer, very practical, and a big worrier. I skirted around or provided light-touch descriptions of day-to-day matters that might concern my parents. I knew I had pushed my father's worry buttons when a letter arrived in his handwriting rather than my mother's.

Dad was onto the matter of safe water supplies soon after my arrival in the country. In one of several letters meant to reassure him, I explained, "I boil and filter all drinking water. We have a good well— protected and uncontaminated as far as we know." I did not explain that the well was hand dug, shallow, and unlined, nor did I mention the lack of testing for well-water contaminants.

My father read between the lines of my skimpy descriptions. He kept returning to the question of safe water. I tried worry suppressant responses. "We are very careful to boil and filter our water. When I'm working in the villages, I take a large flask of water with me. I'm practising what I preach." All this was true, but I did not disclose related matters like eating utensils that were washed with contaminated water when we ate in the villages.

I left out descriptions of serious potable water challenges: severe shortages in the season leading up to the rains, and high rates of gastroenteritis due to groundwater runoff. I did not disclose my roommate's severe episode of dysentery or my bouts of giardia. I made no mention of the chemical contamination of water we observed in a few villages where the pesticide Malathion was sprinkled in streams to kill fish that were sold for human consumption.

In a letter home, I described my first episode of malaria as a "mild case". It was mild because I was diagnosed and treated quickly and appropriately. In fact, my malaria experience was pretty awful and landed me in bed for a few days. I did not explain that I had had falciparum malaria (the most common type of malaria in Sierra Leone) that can lead to cerebral malaria ... too much information. I was mum on two subsequent rounds of malaria—avoiding parental worry-triggers.

There were lengthy delays between letters sent and received, even when the post did go through. By the time one of my letters reached Canada, I was dealing with the next challenge. This left my parents fretting over outdated incidents. Communication delays brought out the worst of retrospective worrying.

The first two years I was in Sierra Leone, no international or intercity phone connections were in place. The Sisters used a ham radio for urgent communication with Freetown, like confirming when a vaccine shipment had arrived. External telecommunications in the capital improved in 1980 after the President of Sierra Leone offered to host the international meeting of the Organization of African Unity in Freetown. President Siaka Stevens was installed as Chairman. Rumour was that Heads of State from other African countries had refused to attend unless international phone lines were available. Their demands reflected a predilection towards political coups when national leaders went abroad.

For the most part, the international phone lines did not provide better communication for those living up-country. However, the new infrastructure offered an enticing reason to go to Freetown. The possibility of calling home was a perk, although timing did not always coincide with days when telephone operators were working.

I initiated one call with my mother during my third year in the country. It was highly unsatisfactory. I phoned home, out-of-the-blue, having come to Freetown unexpectedly. The call lasted all of six minutes before the operator cut us off. It took my mother a minute or two to get over the shock of hearing my voice. We kept talking over each other. I tried to quell her fear that I was calling because of a personal emergency. I did not phone home from Freetown again. Letters were a more satisfactory, albeit constrained, means of conversing with family. Retro-worrying remained their unfortunate consequence.

A Year Back in Canada

When I returned to Canada for graduate school in 1981, my family assumed I was coming home for good. Instead, I announced that I had a fellowship that would allow me to return to Sierra Leone after a year of graduate studies. I was thrilled; my family was not.

I settled into graduate school with enthusiasm. My closest affiliations were with international students from low- and middle-income countries who were part of the International Clinical Epidemiology Network and registered in the same graduate program as me. Several of these students became regular study buddies; my global health research interests aligned with theirs.

With funding from CIDA, McMaster University had a faculty member on secondment in Fourah Bay College, where he was setting up a community health department. Several faculty in my graduate department had been to Sierra Leone and Serabu. I had accompanied them to several villages. This was a bonus. Some faculty in my department had firsthand knowledge of the setting for my proposed thesis topic.

I geared graduate studies towards my interests in low-income countries. While living in Canada, I was comfortably operating in an international bubble. The year was more like a hiatus from my work in Sierra Leone than a re-entry experience.

CHAPTER 20
RESEARCH PLANS

I settled on TBAs as the focus for my thesis. Conversations with these primary health care workers about their challenges and successes echoed in my mind. I frequently told TBA stories when I shared anecdotes with family and friends.

I had a basic understanding of factors influencing the work of granny-midwives in Mende villages, knowledge I considered requisite for a culturally-informed study. The question of how to scale-up TBA training in Sierra Leone perplexed.

I had read preliminary appraisals of the government TBA training that were completed in 1980. Access to published literature was a novelty. When I travelled to Ottawa to assist with Cuso International orientation sessions, I spent time in Ottawa's International Development Research Centre (IDRC) library. I scoured evaluation reports of TBA training programs from different parts of the world, looking for ideas.

Ongoing controversies concerning TBA training and debates about whether or not upgrading a traditional cadre of midwives reduced maternal and neonatal mortality rates caught my attention. I was astonished to learn that TBAs had been out-lawed in a few low-income countries. Some other governments were urging women to seek maternity care exclusively from auxiliary or professionally trained health care workers, while silent regarding the roles of TBAs.

A few well-designed studies had examined the effectiveness of TBA training. Evaluations that had estimated training costs for government or communities were sparse. The question of how to achieve large-scale coverage of TBA training had been superficially addressed.

I was convinced that TBA training programs in Sierra Leone were on the right path. Dr. Williams and Sister Hilary recognized TBAs as resolute health providers with multi-generational roots. Both thought training TBAs would improve maternal and newborn care, reducing morbidity and mortality rates. Important inroads on TBA training had been made through Sierra Leone's country-wide government initiative and Serabu's training. By December 1981, 631 TBAs had received government training.[27] However, it would be years, and many maternal and neonatal deaths later, before either training would reach TBAs in all villages.

I kept coming back to the question of coverage—how to train more TBAs, more quickly, in more villages? Neither the government's nor Serabu Hospital's TBA training could be scaled-up faster without more registered nurse-midwives to do the training. That professional cadre was a scarce resource. The supervision of trained TBAs was another constraint. The government's appraisal of TBA training suggested that MCH aides might help supervise trained TBAs, but this was not yet policy.

TBA training programs of Serabu Hospital and government were distinguishable by their coverage assumptions. Government training aimed to increase the number of villages with at least one trained TBA, country-wide. TBAs had to travel to provincial or district headquarters for a concentrated three-week training period. Not all TBAs were willing or able to do so. Serabu staff trained all women recognized by their communities as TBAs. Training took place in the villages where the grannies lived. Numerous visits were required to complete the lessons. The catchment area was a single chiefdom.

Serabu's approach yielded a high concentration of trained TBAs in each village, but a slower rate of village coverage. While the government program reached more villages faster, training a single TBA from a village did not jive with the cultural threads of *Bundu* Society that bound TBAs together in their midwifery practice.

TBAs who successfully completed either training were given a signed certificate. Each TBA in the government program received a World Health Organization birth kit on graduation. The small aluminum box contained a rubber ground sheet, forceps and scissors to cut the cord, cord ties, and gauze and alcohol to dress the cord. I wasn't sure if those items got used. I had met a few government-trained TBAs in villages. Graduates were proud of their kits, displaying them like hard-won trophies while complaining that kit supplies were not replaced by government.

I did not think the Ministry of Health would be amenable to changes in its TBA training approach nor was it my place to suggest alterations. I was pretty sure Sister Hilary would be open to adjusting Serabu's TBA training to increase its coverage rate. Sister Hilary and I had discussed MCH aides as an appropriate worker for this role.

Preparing MCH aides to train all TBAs in their catchment areas was the essence of what I called the hybrid TBA training. There was a hitch. MCH aides were government workers and not under the authority of Serabu Hospital.

I had my thesis topic. I laid out detailed plans for a study to compare the cost-effectiveness of two TBA training initiatives, the existing government program and the hybrid training that would involve MCH aides rather than professional nurse-midwives as front-line TBA trainers. The hybrid approach could more rapidly scale-up TBA training, while increasing its local accessibility for all granny midwives who assisted with deliveries. I hypothesized that hybrid training would strengthen referral chains by building trust and respect between MCH aides and TBAs. I planned to include a set of control villages whose TBAs would receive no training. My research proposal was deemed methodologically robust and ethically sound by McMaster faculty. I successfully defended my design thesis in August 1982.

I had not checked out my research plans with Sierra Leonean officials. I had plenty of practical excuses: tight timelines to complete my thesis, the unreliable postal service, and the challenges of international phone calls. Deep down, I worried that my request to do the study might be rejected by government authorities. I convinced myself that I'd make a more persuasive case for the study once I was back in the country where I was pretty sure I'd have Sister Hilary's support. I'd need her guidance too.

While I knew what protocols had to be followed to obtain the permission of traditional leaders for community work, I was unfamiliar with the steps required to get government approval for my study. In my thesis, I wrote that one month would be enough time to get permission to proceed.

CHAPTER 21
READY FOR RESEARCH

I was excited to return to Sierra Leone with my TBA study plan and newly minted research skills. My arrival in Freetown was unremarkable. Navigating what had once been a bewildering customs' check and baggage retrieval process at Lungi airport was straightforward.

Despite the familiar setting and predictable airport procedures, everything else seemed different. My CIDA fellowship would cover my living expenses and some research costs. However, I had no job, no community health nurse tutor status, and none of the safeguards I had taken for granted as a CUSO volunteer. I fretted about getting government approval for my independent study.

I needed a lot of goodwill. I would draw on my networks and contacts. At least I had a temporary place to stay. The Sisters at Serabu Hospital had agreed to accommodate me on the hospital compound, for the short-term.

Sister Fidelma Finch met me in Freetown for lunch the day after I arrived. She was an Irish social scientist based at Serabu. She had completed McMaster's Design, Measurement, and Evaluation graduate program the year before me. I found her serious in demeanour, but kind and compassionate in our friendship. We had collaborated on evaluation projects. It was reassuring to see her. I was eager to catch up on her work and hear local stories that rang with familiarity. Sitting on the patio of the only Chinese restaurant in the country, we tucked into sweet and sour chicken. My appetite was off; our meal choice was a metaphor for how I was feeling.

It felt cathartic to share my worries about getting government permission for my TBA study. This was the first time I had verbalized my concerns. I did not expect the overwhelming sense of homesickness and trepidation that coursed through my body and mind as I chatted with Sister Fidelma. I attributed my emotions to jet-lag and exhaustion. I had defended my thesis two weeks before. A whirlwind of pre-departure activities had followed. My unpleasant feelings involved more than physical fatigue. Time with my family in Vancouver had been too short. My completed master's degree was barely under my belt. No longer consumed with finishing my thesis, researcher-imposter thoughts were creeping in. I was over-whelmed by the reality of conducting my ambitious study, which up to that point had been a paper exercise.

Research unknowns and hurdles lay ahead. I had ten months of funding to complete the fieldwork. The brash confidence I had conveyed regarding the feasibility of my study during my thesis defence had evaporated. A dark and anguished thought engulfed me. Coming back to Sierra Leone had been a bad choice—or worse, a stupid mistake.

When I awoke the next morning, my usual sense of optimism had started to return. I did have connections and mentors in the country. I could consult with others who had evaluation and research exper-tise, including Sierra Leoneans who had completed the same gradu-ate program at McMaster before me. And in my heart of hearts, I was convinced my study topic was important. I had returned to do more than a research project. I wanted to give back to the TBAs, who had captivated me with their midwifery work during my years as a CUSO volunteer. My inner voice cajoled. Maybe doing the study could make a difference for some TBAs and the village women they served.

I headed to Serabu to complete the preparatory work for my research alongside colleagues I knew. I shuttled back and forth between Serabu, Freetown, and Bo, meeting with government offi-cials at national and provincial levels to explain my study and seek permission to start. My status at Serabu Hospital had become that of a dislocated, temporary visitor.

Bo-Pujehun Project

My plans had a new wrinkle. Sister Hilary had recently moved to take up a position in Bo. She was employed on a local contract with the German Agency for Technical Cooperation (GTZ). Sister Hilary was the Program Manager for the health and nutrition components of a new and ambitious bilateral and integrated initiative, the Bo-Pujehun Rural Development Project, which everyone unofficially called the Bo-Pujehun project. Health and nutrition operated alongside other programs in agriculture, fisheries, adult literacy, community development, primary education, rural water supplies, and roads. Sister Hilary was working closely with the Ministry of Health's senior provincial team. Her counterpart was the Medical Officer of Health for the Southern Province.

Inception details for the Bo-Pujehun project included plans to evaluate its health impact. Baseline data collection in the two districts was the first step. Sister Hilary asked if I'd advance this work while I waited for the government's go-ahead to conduct my TBA study. I eagerly took this on.

My research seemed to be a good fit with the project's goals of reducing maternal and infant morbidity and mortality rates. I surmised the opportunity to assist with baseline evaluation might also solve a problem. I needed to launch the hybrid portion of my TBA study in at least two districts and in multiple chiefdoms in order to have enough MCH aides and study villages to meet sample size requirements. I raised the possibility of using Bo and Pujehun Districts as study sites for the TBA hybrid training and control villages with Sister Hilary. She was keen.

Permission to conduct the overall comparative study had to be granted by Dr. Williams, the CMO. The new TBA training role for MCH aides would have to be negotiated and approved. I also needed approval to attend and evaluate the government's next TBA training in the Southern Province.

The post-TBA training follow-up period for data collection was short for both arms of the study. I would shave off a chunk of time needed to wrap up the whole study by doing the analysis and report writing back in Canada. My timelines were tight. Nevertheless, plans seemed to be falling into place. From my initial discussions with Sister Hilary and government authorities, approval for my TBA study seemed imminent.

CHAPTER 22
RELOCATING TO BO

Sister Hilary suggested I move to Bo. She invited me to temporarily stay with the Holy Rosary Sisters until alternate lodging was found. The convent was quiet, secure, and by Western standards, fittingly Spartan. My room had a cot, bureau, night stand, and a small wooden desk and chair. We had light as Bo was electrified. That is to say the convent was connected to the city's electrical grid.

After a few weeks of calling the convent home, Sister Hilary announced that she had arranged for me to move in with Judith, a Welsh lab technician who worked with the Medical Research Council (MRC) laboratory. I was pleased to be in more permanent accommodation. Judith seemed content, in a high-strung sort of way, to acquire a roommate. Her work focused on the prevention of onchocerciasis. I anticipated unsavoury dinner conversations about excised "oncho" nodules that Judith and her staff were examining in the lab.

My new abode was up-scale compared to my living quarters in Serabu. It was a good-sized bungalow with a side veranda, where we ate breakfast and enjoyed the birds, flowering plants, and passion fruit vines in our small garden. The house had two bedrooms, a bathroom with a flush toilet and bathtub, and a spacious, well-furnished reception room. The indoor kitchen had an electric fridge and gas stove. Yaya, our cook, used a small outdoor kitchen for food preparation and clean-up.

Our one air conditioner was in my bedroom. On stifling nights when Bo's power was on, Judith and I shared my room. The floor of the house was tiled and cool underfoot. Breezes flowed and insects gained entry through slatted cinder blocks on the outdoor wall of a wide hallway. A ceiling fan in the reception room kept bugs at bay.

A cement-block fence had been built around the perimeter of our narrow yard. Embedded shards of glass discouraged would-be thieves from scaling the structure, but made the property look prison-like. Our watchman, Pa Bockarie, manned the metal gate that secured Judith's car in our short driveway. Pa was kindly and proud of his younger wife and nine kids. His school-age children dropped by to spend time with him some afternoons. Pa had been a house painter. He grew vegetables in our garden for his family. He was a reliable security guard, willing to take on extra work assignments.

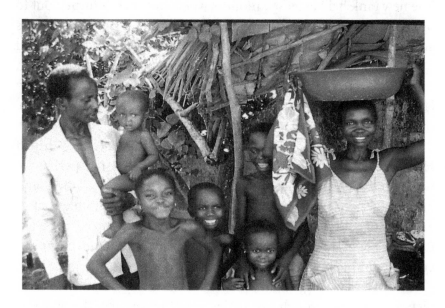

Pa Bockarie (our watchman) with his wife and younger children under the lean-to shelter that he built in the garden of the house where Judith and I lived (Bo, 1984).

I never felt insecure or threatened in Bo, although we had one incident when someone used a long pole to try and lift a few items out of Judith's room. Her windows were open and Bockarie was away. The thief's pole was barely long enough to reach through the gate and past the window frame. He only managed to disturb Judith's bedding.

We did not get to know our local neighbours very well. Judith and I spent a lot of time in the field. However, we did have quite a few international guests, in particular those associated with the MRC lab, including the Director's teenagers.

The flush toilet seriously stressed our water conservation efforts during the dry season. There weren't many water-delivery trucks in Bo. Our roof-level water tank was small, so even when it got filled, the supply barely lasted a few days. After months of complaining, our landlord agreed to have a much larger, cement holding-tank built on the property.

Judith and I were initially pleased with the home improvement. The new tank held at least a month's worth of water. It turned out to be a dismal failure. We called it the soaking tank because its walls acted like a sponge, absorbing and evaporating precious liquid before we had a chance to use it. We suspected the cement had been mixed improperly and started up a new litany of complaints. Our landlord refused to acknowledge the problem. Shortly after I left Bo, the tank collapsed.

Because the MRC lab was run under the auspices of the British High Commission, living with Judith came with other perks. We occasionally used the British consular mail bag to get letters and packages home. We enjoyed imported dairy products like butter and cheese and received invitations to stay at the home of the High Commissioner in Freetown when he was away. The volunteer experience of working in international development was socially stratified.

Through my tangential MRC connection, I ordered a Raleigh bicycle part-way through my final year in the country. The bike was delivered to Freetown via the High Commissioner's mail bag and to our house by the High Commissioner himself. I put the Flying Pigeon bicycle fiasco behind me. I used my new bike to get to and from work and loved the new-found freedom it gave me around town.

Pa Bockarie to the Rescue

When I moved to Bo's urban environment, I reckoned that snake incidents in my home were behind me. This was not so. Pa Bockarie had spotted cobras in our yard. Nevertheless, Judith and I believed that the indoor areas of our house were impervious to snakes. We were wrong.

I was sorting and packing for an international trip. All of my belongings—clothes, books, and work papers were strewn across the floor and furniture of my bedroom. Taking a break from this chore, I was walking towards the kitchen when I spotted a thin, green snake heading for my bedroom. I assumed the worst. Vipers were deadly poisonous. I screamed "snake." Judith and I beetled outside. Pa was at the ready. He had a long stick perched by the lean-to where he spent part of his days. He rushed in, prepared to attack.

The snake had vanished. It had probably slithered into my bedroom and found a hiding place amidst the clutter. Pa would have to locate the reptile by removing clothing items with his long stick. Judith and I huddled like cowards outside the house. Bockarie began the tiresome extraction process. Fifteen minutes later, Pa's shouts signalled success. He'd glimpsed the snake's tail flicking under the buffet beside my bedroom door and clobbered it. The snake turned out to be harmless. Nevertheless, Bockarie crossly explained, "*You geh for white em, so you no go loss em.*" A perfect Krio expression that means you have to watch the snake, so you don't lose sight of it.

CHAPTER 23

SEEKING PERMISSION AND A RAGING GRANNY

On Sept 28, 1982, Dr. Williams told me that my TBA study would be valuable for Sierra Leone. I received her verbal approval to proceed with the study on October 12, 1982. She asked me to keep her informed. I was set to go, relieved that obtaining necessary approval had been so straightforward.

Government TBA Training

My first order of business was to attend the government's TBA training, scheduled to take place in Moyamba District in November. Sister Samai, a stocky, matter-of-fact nurse-midwife with a wide smile was in charge. She invited me to attend the admission interviews of TBA candidates and their three-week training. I needed temporary accommodation.

Fortunately, a volunteer had been posted to teach at Moyamba's secondary school. She had an extra room in her home and agreed to let me stay with her. I had worried that she'd not be on speaking terms with me. I had attended her Cuso International orientation and been assigned to repack her luggage since she was well over the weight limit. I had been the bad-cop, stipulating that she'd have to leave behind some of her favourite shoes (she had packed more than a dozen pairs) and her foodstuff stash (dried carrots, onions, and spices). She had been miffed with my directives. We put that behind us, and she welcomed me into her home.

Interviews to select TBAs for training were conducted by the provincial health sisters in the district government office. Even I felt out of place in that formal environment. TBAs were interviewed in Krio or Mende. The sisters translated some of the Mende responses for me. I concentrated on the TBAs' facial expressions and body language.

The provincial health sisters tried to identify TBAs who would benefit most from the training. They were friendly and direct, putting TBAs at ease with light-hearted talk. TBAs gained their composure as they earnestly described their midwifery work and why they wanted to attend training.

The selection process screened out wannabe TBAs with little or no midwifery experience. The trainers delved into applicants' relationships with their local communities, their interest in learning new skills, and personal motivations for applying. A few applicants were cagey about their actual hands-on delivery experience, before disclosing that they were close relatives of Chiefs who wanted them to get a government certificate and take up midwifery.

One of the younger candidates was deemed a misfit. She had a strong aptitude for midwifery. However, with seven years of formal education, she was over-qualified. The sisters encouraged her to seek admission to MCH aide training.

I was surprised by TBAs' willingness to disclose incidents of difficult deliveries and bad outcomes. I was left with strong impressions of traditional midwives who operated in parallel with, rather than in conjunction with, the government's obstetrical care system.

Nearly 30 TBAs were invited to attend training in a government building adjacent to Moyamba Hospital. We were far from the *Bundu* bush. I found the artificial classroom setting disconcerting.

Small groups of TBAs were sent to the maternity unit to observe deliveries and the examination of placentas for abnormalities. TBAs chatted among themselves as they returned to the classroom. Some expressed concerns regarding testy relationships with hospital staff. Trainers acknowledged that solutions needed to be found. I hoped the TBAs' forays into the delivery room had seeded positive relationships.

Trainers explained and reviewed course content, using familiar analogies (fallopian tubes and ovaries look like palm wine gourds strung from either end of a carrying stick) and role plays. I was surprised so much time was spent showing TBAs how to use the forceps and scissors in their birth kits. While every one of those TBAs plaited hair at eye-catching speed, they had no muscle memory for using either scissors or forceps. Even after hours of practising, TBAs' handling of the tools looked cumbersome. I was skeptical they would use the instruments during a village delivery. I reckoned more emphasis should have been placed on sterilizing traditional cord-cutting items. I was an observer and kept those ruminations to myself.

A Step Backwards

I planned to hold a train-the-trainer workshop for MCH aides after Christmas and began work on the curriculum. Then, on December 13, I received a letter from Dr. Williams. She withdrew permission for that part of the study, citing policy considerations and the need for a thorough review by the Ministry of a program to train MCH aides as TBA trainers.

I made an urgent appointment to see her. Two days later, I travelled to Freetown. The CMO was away, so I was invited to meet with the head of the MCH Division, Dr. Gba Kamara. I made no headway getting approval reinstated for MCH aides to be prepared as TBA trainers, but left his office impressed by a chance encounter with a trained TBA.

Raging Granny

As I presented my case to prepare MCH aides as TBA trainers, a government-trained TBA burst through the door. She had a young teenage boy reluctantly in tow. The Commissioner followed, apologetically muttering that the TBA had insisted she must see the Department Head immediately. Dr. Gba Kamara invited the granny to stay. Cryptic greetings were exchanged while the TBA caught her breath. Mama Mariatu had taken a taxi from the outskirts of Freetown. She was an older woman, and she was in a rage.

Speaking in Krio, Mama launched into her list of complaints. She had sent the teenager to the Ministry offices twice to get supplies for her delivery kit. The alcohol, cord ties, and gauze used to be dispensed on the first Wednesday of the month. Both times that she sent for supplies, the boy returned empty-handed.

Prior to her TBA training, people paid her in kind or with cash for deliveries. *Belly women* now say the granny is being paid by the government because she was trained by the government. She no longer gets anything for her work and to make matters worse, there are no supplies. The day before, she assisted nurses in a cottage hospital to deliver a woman who was having a difficult labour. These nurses had other supplies like gloves, which are not in her birth kit; she would like to have gloves too. The pregnant women who went to the cottage hospital had to pay Le 10. Mama Mariatu got no *small-small* payment for her work. So she had decided to come and see the Head herself.

Catching her breath and calming a bit, she reached into her bag to pull out her framed TBA certificate and delivery book. She was proud of her training.

Dr. Gba Kamara explained the problem with supplies and suggested that the TBA ask pregnant women to pay for their deliveries. Mama Mariatu was about to restart her rant. She was adamant, stating she had *"too much sorry heart for dem belly women"* to ask them directly for compensation.

This granny saw and lived the cycle of poverty that existed in her community. Asking for payment would break her covenant with the pregnant women she served. The Director extended his thanks to this TBA for her services and offered well-meaning platitudes. Mama Mariatu was courteously dismissed.

No solution had been found. Dr. Gba Kamara looked dejected. His boss was the architect of the government TBA training. He was aware that the issues raised by this TBA could erode goodwill that had been built between TBAs and government nurse-midwives during training.

Mama Mariatu was determined not to undermine the long-standing relationship she had with her community. I hoped she left the exchange emboldened. She had asserted a subtle power and explained the concerns of granny midwives to someone who held the levers for change in government. She had eloquently voiced the realities of vulnerable women in her community. Training had bolstered her midwifery skills and led her to the Director's office, where she had advocated for pregnant women.

Although heartened by the TBA's intervention, permission for my study had not been reinstated. Dr. Gba Kamara indicated the matter required further consideration by the National Maternal and Child Health Advisory Committee. Nothing could happen until after the holidays. I left the office worried and dejected.

Study Ramifications

Looking back, I had not appreciated the policy implications of my TBA research study. It is generous to describe my assumptions about proceeding with this work as naïve. My suggestion that the roles of MCH aides be expanded to include TBA training had been met with skepticism. Who would supervise this work? Were MCH aides up to the task with only 18 months of basic training? Existing government TBA training was led by professional nurse-midwives—most with international qualifications. What were the short- and long-term costs of this alternate training plan?

I was mum on all of these important system matters. My omissions were red flags, indicating that my training idea was ill-informed if not flawed. When I look back at my research plans, my blatant silences are downright embarrassing.

Unlike Sister Hilary, who had dedicated her lifetime medical work to Sierra Leone, I was a bit player. At best, I was a transient and must have been viewed as one of those foreign nationals who comes and goes with their helicopter research. While I had worked in Serabu for a few years, I was brand new on the government scene. I had no street-creds as a researcher.

Worse, the government had recently completed an extensive evaluation of their TBA training, examining knowledge, attitudes, and practices. I was asking to conduct a study comparing the existing government program with a new training approach. Wasn't this premature and duplicative? At best, I must have been viewed as impudent, audacious, and inexperienced by Dr. Williams—and I wasn't even qualified as a midwife.

Awaiting Permission

I was in the midst of a tortuous, eight-month period, seeking and re-seeking study permissions. I was nearly halfway through my allotted time for the study and restarting the process of getting permission for the hybrid training arm of my research. I felt morose. My naïveté had fuelled my optimism. I had grossly underestimated how long it would take to get permission. This quandary weighed heavily on me over Christmas. I had no source of funding for any additional time in Sierra Leone when my fellowship ended in June.

Sister Hilary was a huge support, confidant, and guide for me during this prolonged period of waiting. She had an excellent working relationship with Dr. Williams and acted as liaison, explaining the relevance of my proposed research and advocating for permission to be granted.

My enthusiasm and get-at-it attitude waned, as the back-and-forth research permission question continued. On January 24, 1983, I received exciting news. The CMO had verbally re-approved data collection for my TBA study, as long as it was undertaken within the context of the Bo-Pujehun project. Written permission was forthcoming. Yet, explicit approval for what I considered to be the novel element of my project, training MCH aides to be TBA trainers was outstanding.

Given the withering time I had to complete the study, I'd need to have the MCH aide training ready to go, if and when Ministry approval was granted. I teamed up with a British physician, Dr. Rosemary McMahon, whose husband headed up the MRC laboratory. Rosemary had joined Sister Hilary's primary health care team.

She was a gifted educator who guided my MCH aide curriculum development efforts.

By February, I had a curriculum to train MCH aides but no written permission to proceed. Sister Hilary interceded. She called Dr. Williams on a day when the inter-city phone in her office was working. She explained that I was just looking, in a scientific way, into whether or not the methods of TBA training worked. A new measure of hesitation crept into the conversation. The CMO indicated that others had reservations about my project. Dr. Williams was concerned that the study would involve re-deploying MCH aides. This was a policy matter and required further appraisal. My heart sank, the permission process was going backwards.

On March 5, Sister Hilary was called to a meeting with national and provincial Ministry of Health bigwigs to discuss the hybrid TBA training. They gave their verbal okay. Dr. Williams insisted that training MCH aides to train TBAs was a contingency arrangement. Her caution may have reflected swelling sentiments in World Health Organization circles that auxiliary nurse-midwives rather than TBAs were the cadre needed to improve maternal and child health care.

Dr. Williams still had outstanding questions. Would certificates be provided and, if so, would these be equivalent to those issued to TBAs who completed the standard government training? Which government health sister should be in charge of the new MCH aide training? What were the appropriate lines of communication for this work? I awaited written permission.

CHAPTER 24
BASELINE SURVEY FIELDWORK

In December 1982, I was busy preparing for the Bo-Pujehun baseline survey. The work was a good distraction from the permission-granting process for my TBA study. I had lots of experience with small-scale community needs' assessments that Serabu's public health team had conducted in several dozen villages in Bumpe, Magbosi, and Mattru Chiefdoms while I was a CUSO volunteer. The baseline survey was different. It would be launched in over 500 villages. Interviewers were government employees rather than Serabu's nursing students. My working relationship with EDCU assistants was murky, given my unofficial status with the Bo-Pujehun project.

The survey work was a tall order. EDCU assistants would be conducting interviews in dispersed villages. Much of their work would be solo, with little on-site supervision. If they ran into trouble, they'd be on their own.

I worked with government staff to finalize questionnaires, plan training for interviewers, and organize a pilot of household interviews. Ministry officials prepared letters to introduce EDCU assistants to Chiefs.

Selecting villages for the baseline study was a tedious paper and pencil exercise completed by Ministry staff. A list of all 2,100 villages in Bo and Pujehun Districts from the 1974 census were divided into groups (sampling strata) according to size (1-199 versus 200-2,000) and proximity to a peripheral health unit (3 miles or less, more than 3 miles). A random sample of villages was selected from each strata. Enumerators were assigned to geographic clusters of study villages.

Printing

In January 1983, we were ready to train interviewers, conduct the pilot, and launch EDCU assistants into the field for data collection. And then we ran into the first big hiccup.

I had anticipated printing delays. Record-keeping books such as patient registers were in increasingly short supply. I had seen this firsthand. At Moyamba Hospital, I asked to review annual records of newborns admitted and deliveries attended. I was told the records had been sent to Freetown for security reasons. No duplicate records existed in Moyamba because staff had no paper. The in-charge clerk explained that no records had been kept at the hospital for months. They had no forms and central stores had none in stock. The clerk was working on the problem. He had placed a piggy bank on his desk to raise funds for stationary; a 1980s version of crowdfunding.

I sent master copies of the questionnaires to the government printers in Freetown, thinking this would be an efficient means to get the job done. It was anything but that, as I vented in my journal. Printing delays were blamed on the lack of paper and power blackouts. These problems were reverberating through other aspects of my work and home life, and whittling away my patience.

Journal Entries

January to March 1983

Bo

January 26th

> We've been waiting for weeks. The questionnaires aren't back from Freetown. Electricity has been off in the capital for several days.

January 30th

> I made yet another phone call to ask about the baseline question-naires. Latest news from the printing office is that there is not enough paper to run them off. This means that the thorough job EDCU staff just completed of notifying Chiefs in nine villages

about the upcoming survey is of little use and inadvertently has been downright misleading.

I can't get out to a small team of interviewers who have been conducting other work in Tikonko. There's no petrol in Bo and no transport available. So much for supportive supervision.

Judith and I have no water at home. Bo's electricity has been off for three days. We go to our dependable Lebanese restaurant, the Rio, to get something to eat. It's closed. A sign on the door states the obvious: *Power no deh.*

February 1st

The questionnaire forms in Freetown have still not been printed; power blackouts is the reason given. A colleague suggests that we run them off using stencils. We're holding off on this option. I'm worried the Gestetner machine in the Ministry office would grind to a halt with such demanding copying requirements. Getting the Gestetner repaired might take weeks or months.

There is a bit of good news from Freetown. According to my German colleague, who spoke to the manager in charge of printing, 18,000 sheets of paper are now available. He urged the manager to start the printing immediately so he can bring some of the questionnaires to my office when he returns to Bo tomorrow.

February 2nd

My German colleague arrived back in Bo. Still no questionnaires.

February 4th

One of the provincial health sisters comes into Sister Hilary's office asking for paper to run off the annual under-five clinic figures. Paper *no deh.*

The EDCU supervisor is looking for paper to print a questionnaire about the cholera outbreak in Taninahun. Two adults have already died. They also need drugs and asked for 2,000 doses of tetracycline, syringes, and IV fluids. The Bo-Pujehun project office has no such supplies.

Norman, the Ministry's "Gestetner man" asks Sister Hilary for medicine for his gripping abdominal pain. He'll probably be off sick for a few days. No one else knows how to run the machine.

Semi-good news today. Half of the questionnaires have now been printed. They are sitting in the government printing office. For reasons unknown, the project's driver in Freetown was unable to collect them. It doesn't look like Mariba, the provincial government driver, can help. He comes into Sister Hilary's office with a very swollen wrist, the result of his having fought for three gallons of petrol in the cue.

Late February

No electricity in Bo during working hours. Judith and I are down to our last gallon of water. The power comes on for a few hours at 8 PM. There were student riots in Freetown today to protest petrol shortages. Primary and secondary school students are striking and threatening to damage the President's car tomorrow if nothing is done.

March 1st

The Provincial Medical Officer of Health has been stuck in Bo. He's waited two days to travel while his driver tries to get petrol. The phone lines to Freetown have been down for four days. Ministry staff are using the radio for inter-office communications.

The printed questionnaires arrived in early March. I wasn't sure whether my dogged persistence or forcibly imposed forbearance had served me better.

Classroom Training

In March, I was fully occupied training EDCU assistants for the Bo-Pujehun survey. My patience was running short, my enthusiasm dulled. I lost my temper with trainees more than once when they asked me, yet again, to clarify payment for their per diems and overnight allowances. It rankled that I was doing the training work and heavy-lifting on the baseline survey with no salary. I reminded myself that the Bo-Pujehun project was paying my rent, and my CIDA scholarship funds were more than enough for me to live on.

Logistics

Managing logistics for fieldwork was like a Snakes and Ladders game with starts, stops, standstills, and reversals. Advance preparations could create a make-it or break-it scenario for interviewers. On-the-spot modifications to plans were frequently required.

Study villages in Bo and Pujehun Districts were grouped according to geographic proximity. EDCU assistants travelled in *poda-podas* to Chiefdom headquarters, where they sorted out routes to study villages with the assistance of Paramount Chiefs and Speakers. Local escorts accompanied interviewers to villages that had to be reached by foot.

Senior Ministry personnel prepared letters to inform Chiefdom and village leaders about the surveys and to obtain permission to proceed. Letters were written in English. We never knew what translation vagaries undermined well-crafted messages.

There was no guarantee that hand-delivered notices regarding upcoming data collection got to the right people. Selecting suitable dates was one-sided guesswork, layered on the uncertainty of transportation and unpredictable fuel supplies. Precise scheduling was nonsensical.

EDCU workers carried two official letters. An introductory letter described who the worker was and the nature of his work. A formally-worded letter was addressed to the Paramount Chief and requested permission for the enumerator to complete the survey in his or her chiefdom. A cascade of permission requests and approvals or refusals followed.

Government employees were sometimes viewed with skepticism or hostility. EDCU assistants could be spurned and find themselves treading in the territory of fractious relationships. Ministry authorization of the study occasionally put EDCU assistants in a bad spot. As government workers, they inadvertently represented prior wrongs and broken promises. Discouraged interviewers reported instances when Chiefs denied them permission to proceed because of earlier incidents.

> We don't think our women will come this time [to participate in the study] because you government people always come here and lie to us. Government people came here and removed our blood, each person, one to two pints, and told us that they were going to send us medicines. Until now, they are still not coming with the medicines.

> There was a time when a certain fellow came here and lied to us. Just to collect 50 cents from each person, saying that the government sent him to do so. We don't think government workers will fool us again.

> Mr. Government man, we are not ready for you because you government people all the time lie to us saying that you will make our roads. The roads you [the government] made last are the ones you were walking on [to get to our village].

Getting the Work Done

Advance notification did not ensure that authorities were *on seat* when an interviewer arrived. Chiefs and Speakers had other responsibilities like court cases, village disputes, crises, and burials. High-ranking individuals within male or female Secret Societies had related duties. Most were also farmers. Return trips were sometimes required before EDCU assistants got permission to proceed.

Interviewers worked around the uncertainty of permissions granted or postponed. They reported a plethora of scheduling machinations. Enumerators were ultra-adept at adjusting work plans and moving back and forth between villages to obtain permission from the right authorities to complete survey work.

Mr. Conteh, an EDCU assistant, filed reports describing the types of challenges he encountered: waiting for a Chief to return from a trip, pausing for TBAs to attend a pregnant woman in labour, and delaying work due to illness and deaths. In a nutshell, village life happens.

> I departed Bo for Gerihun to report to the Paramount Chief. Arriving at Gerihum, [I was told that] the Paramount Chief had gone to Lunsar to attend eye clinic. I was referred to the Chiefdom Speaker at Baoma. I travelled to Baoma and introduced myself to the Speaker, handing over the letter for the Paramount Chief. The Speaker assisted by providing me with an escort to Nyandehun. Arriving, I introduced myself to the Chiefs and explained my mission to their village. While they were trying to inform the TBAs about my visit, sad news was brought that the Chief's wife, who is also a sister of the TBA, had died at the Bo Government Hospital. At this junction, I was asked by the authorities to proceed to another village and call back at their convenient time. (H.S. Conteh, May 1983)

Fieldwork Challenges

Interviewers faced pragmatic difficulties. Some Chiefs were slow to organize food and lodging. Evening work was thwarted when neither lamps nor candles were available. Long bush-walks were exhausting. Injuries occurred. Poisonous snakes were occupational dangers. Interviewers risked getting infectious diseases. Gastroenteritis and malaria were common. EDCU assistants did not receive hazard pay.

I worried most about perilous political situations, which could unexpectedly arise while EDCU assistants were in the field. Several instances of violence jeopardized interviewers' safety. Sister Hilary swiftly travelled to Pujehun to confer with Chiefs after enumerators from three Chiefdoms in that district returned to Bo for safety reasons.

Journal Entry

May 1983

Pujehun District

A Section Chief was killed last week and attempts were made on the Paramount Chief's life. An EDCU assistant came [back to Bo] from Makpele Chiefdom. He was in a village that was under ambush; gunfire was heard. The villagers led him to safety in the coffee bush and sent a group of men out to meet another EDCU assistant on the road and prevent him from coming into the village.

Facing an ambush surpassed the call of duty. Rare as it was, safeguards were near impossible. EDCU assistants' supervisors relied on Chiefs to warn of simmering problems or volatile situations. Local authorities tried to provide a security bubble for government enumerators.

Getting Paid

Even when deployed for fieldwork, EDCU assistants had to make the time-consuming trip back to the Treasurer's office in Bo to collect cash on pay days. Morale dipped when government salaries went unpaid. Strike action was off the table. No pay meant the coffers were empty. EDCU assistants returned to their assigned villages to resume household interviews, worrying about their own families in Bo, hoping the next pay-day scenario would be different.

I finally understood why overnight allowances had been such a point of contention when I trained EDCU assistants. This was the one tangible incentive they received for their arduous work. I found it nothing short of remarkable that assistants completed their surveys.

Sidelined

In late March, 1983 I landed in Serabu Hospital with appendicitis. The timing was awful. Interviewers had just begun baseline data collection. Thankfully, Ministry staff were responsible for field supervision.

Nothing like a week of post-operative recovery to regain perspective on life. I missed the evaluation work. My preoccupying concerns about future career directions was a problem of too many choices. So few of my Sierra Leonean colleagues had the luxury of career options. I recalled conversations with EDCU assistants and stories of their lives I had pieced together. Many bore the financial burden and expectations of extended families, while experiencing the recurring problem of salaries delayed for one or two months. Gainful employment was hard to come by. Some were frustrated in their jobs, having experienced the thrill of being hired as a government employee, followed by long delays in training that left them bored and under-employed. They were eager to contribute, be deployed, and assist with the Expanded Program of Immunization or outbreak management.

Training for the baseline study had given participating EDCU assistants a renewed sense of purpose and augmented their skill sets. While they expected challenging fieldwork conditions, most had welcomed the opportunity to be involved. My career-choice conundrum seemed selfish and paltry.

CHAPTER 25
A GLIMPSE OF HISTORICAL TRAUMAS

A few weeks after my appendectomy, two friends, Jenny and Judith, suggested a short holiday in Shenge over the Easter weekend. We travelled in Jenny's small car.

Shenge is on Sierra Leone's southern coast; its beauty belies its troubled past. Slaves from the West African region were sold and bought on this coastline until the British passed the Slavery Abolition Act in 1833 that made the purchase or ownership of slaves within the British Empire illegal. The juxtaposition of Shenge's tropical paradise of sandy beaches and nearby islands with the historical scars of slave trading was stark and unsettling. I wondered how the locals recounted slavery.

Our temporary abode was the bare-bones government rest house. Twice a day, the Paramount Chief and dispenser had school children deliver us cooked meals. Each was the same, fresh barracuda atop a heaping mound of rice, served on a mauve plastic plate with a big red chili pepper on the side. The meals were scrumptious.

We enjoyed languid swims at a beach near the rest house. I wrote my parents with news of my surgery since I was well on my way to recovery. On a reassurance scale, I botched that correspondence. I omitted post-surgical details, like the spinal headache that laid me flat for a week. Explaining that complication would have involved disclosing the state of anesthetics and empty oxygen tanks at Serabu Hospital. I emphasized my recuperative vacation in Shenge with the long ocean swims and the fresh and tasty barracuda. Months later, my mother explained that my ill-conceived recovery account had caught her attention. "Inglis, isn't barracuda a type of shark?" she had asked my father. Busted.

Plantain Island

On market day, we set out to visit Plantain Island, a bustling fishing community and an historic site with bad karma. Despite the early morning hour, Shenge's beach was buzzing with travellers from the island's flotilla. Mothers with infants and toddlers clutched yellow immunization cards as they headed to clinic. This was a social outing; women had tied their colourful headscarves with extra care.

Men were ready for heavy work. Stripped to the waist, they head-carried large bundles of dried fish to lorries. Young boys unloaded empty jerry cans; some would be filled with water, others with petrol. Well water on the island was brackish, drinking water came from Shenge. Petrol for outboard motors was sold at black market prices. Supplies had to last until the next mid-week trading day.

After haggling, we hired a boat with a sputtering outboard motor for our trip to the island. The boatman charged us Le 11 for one gallon of petrol and Le 4 for transfer service "*waste time*". As we arrived onshore, a young teen, who spoke Krio, offered to show us around. He took us to the far end of the island—a small rock outcropping with scrubby trees, adjoined by a narrow isthmus that flooded at high tide.

Our guide pointed to the remnants of John Newton's house and the one remaining wall of the prison-like barracoon that had been built into the rock. Mr. Newton was an English slave master, himself indentured to a slave owner on Banana Island. He had lived on Plantain Island and run a factory where slaves had been bought and sold by traders who had plied the West African coast. Shivers ran through me as I pictured innocent captives transported in chains, facing inhumane living conditions in the holding pens. This land, on which I freely walked, had been a cruel and evil prison for generations of people my age.

I had questions, but my queries were for an elder, not an adolescent, and so they went unasked. What did parents share with their children and what did schools teach about the history of slavery? Who were the local knowledge keepers of the slave trade? How did the ancestors offer protection against any slave trade *juju* that pulsed in this land? My head reeled.

Our tour guide wandered away. He sensed that we needed time to ourselves.

I dredged up superficial bits of information about the trans-Atlantic slave trade I'd gleaned in high school. Since coming to Sierra Leone, I had learned more about the history of the Creoles and their Canadian connections. The underground railway had brought some emancipated slaves to Nova Scotia. Africville was the area where Black Loyalists from the American Civil War had settled in search of a better life. They had been disappointed by unfilled British promises of land allotments.

My maternal grandparents had lived in Halifax, not far from Africville. I never heard them mention Nova Scotian black settlers. My mother recalled men from Africville driving ox-carts to Halifax on Saturdays to collect food scraps for their pigs. She knew nothing of the 1,000 Nova Scotian black settlers who returned to the area in West Africa that they named Freetown, where they comprised part of the Creole population. I knew no West African slavery stories of family dislocation and fracture or Creoles' accounts of settling or resettling on the African continent.

Slavery had been banned, but its racializing tentacles still ran deep in North America. I flashed back to my brief and disagreeable sense of racial divides in Louisiana. I recalled the burnt-out buildings I had seen in Detroit after the race riots in the late 1960s, the despair that followed Martin King Junior's assassination, and news reports of de-segregation in American schools. This small site on Plantain Island, with its tumbled slave trade remnants, had forged new bridges in my psyche, linking past and present.

I shifted my feet in the sand, sensing the weight of this tragic past. I paused in a woefully inadequate moment of remembrance for the thousands who had been forcibly transported along the West African coast to Sierra Leone's slave trading sites in the 1700s.

I was ashamed of my sparse knowledge fragments concerning this scourge of human migration. Not knowing was not okay. I vowed to read more about slavery, the slave trade, and its intergenerational repercussions when I returned home.

Our young guide returned to continue the informal island tour. My mind flipped back to the present as we retraced our steps, dodging tidal pools. He led us back to the beach that ran alongside the small shanty village. More permanent-looking homes sat in the middle of the island. Temporary lean-to huts provided additional shelter. The predominantly Sherbro community swelled with seasonal Temne residents during the dry season.

Despite its raw beauty, this was not a tourist area. Shad fish was the island's primary trading commodity; everyone bustled with fishing activities. Solo boatmen plied the water in dugout canoes. Fishers worked in unison, casting and heaving nets from plank boats powered by rudimentary sails. Men, women, and children retrieved the catch at the shoreline. Artisanal fishing was a whole-community enterprise.

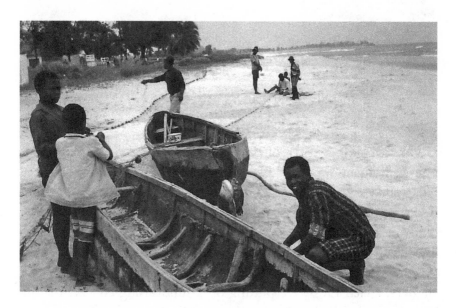

Artisanal fishermen with rustic boats and fishing nets (Plantain Island, 1983). The slave barracoon I visited was at one end of the island.

Older men repaired large fishing nets laid out on the beach. Goats wandered. Women worked through the haze of sooty smoke, rotating fresh catch and dried bonga on large racks, stoking charcoal fires, and packing baskets with smoked fish for transport. All the while, they minded little ones. My friends and I were a distraction. School-age children gathered round, asking us to take their photos. Sand flies bit my ankles.

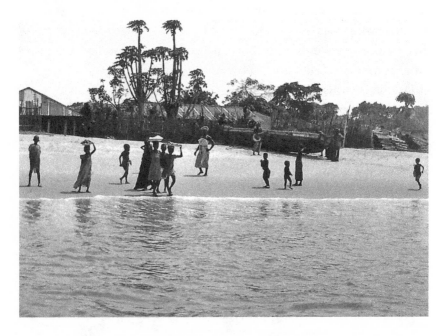

School-age children gathered on beach (Plantain Island, 1983).

One evening, a surge of people streamed past the guest house. The excitement was palpable. A Lebanese man who lived in the village had a private generator and offered a video screening from his living room. We joined dozens of children and adults spilling out from his front veranda, which had become a makeshift theatre. The television blasted at full volume. Bobbing heads vied for viewing positions of the small screen that was barely visible through open shutters. Celebrities were putting on a fundraising concert for the Falkland Islands' crisis. It was otherworldly.

A call to Easter Sunday service in the old church came from a large metal object hanging on a tree branch. An enthusiastic youngster hit it repeatedly with an iron bar; a raucous call to prayer that left my ears ringing. Jenny, Judith, and I were escorted to the front of the small church where we were invited to sit in the choir pew beside the Paramount Chief. This was an honour. Hot, muggy air prolonged the meandering sermon delivered in Krio. Hymns sung in beautiful harmonies punctuated the long service.

The next day, work beckoned. We headed back to Bo. I counted bridges on the first leg of our return trip—75 culverts between Shenge and Sembehun, a 36-mile jaunt. As the self-assigned navigator, I directed Jenny as she drove across the two- and three-log bridge spans. I was in and out of the back seat 20 times for the most treacherous crossings. Our grueling staccato trip home shook us back into reality.

CHAPTER 26
MCH AIDE TRAINING

On April 12, 1983, Sister Hilary arrived back from a trip to Freetown with my long-awaited approval letter in hand. Dr. Williams had granted written permission for my full TBA research study. MCH aide training could proceed. I had booked my flight home for May 28. That gave me six weeks to do the impossible.

I don't know what played out behind the scenes in the ultimate granting of permission for the hybrid portion of my study. It probably helped that a number of senior public health physicians from Sierra Leone had completed the same master's degree that I had at McMaster University. They may have vouched for me. Dr. Victor Cole, who was one of those graduates, had been a strong supporter of my study from the get-go. Whether or not my colleagues' input garnered me a small degree of credibility, I'll never know. I am forever grateful to Dr. Williams for the chance she took on me.

The nine-day workshop for MCH aide trainers was scheduled to run from May 4. Sister Fofana, a petite, cracker-jack public health nurse supervisor, was in charge of the training. Sisters Samai and Scott assisted. The twenty MCH aides who were invited to the workshop came from health centres in Bo and Pujehun Districts. With the list of participating MCH aides and their health centres in hand, I could finally select study villages for the hybrid training evaluation.

I laid large maps of Bo and Pujehun Districts on the floor of my house. Perched on the maps, my eyes and fingers hop-scotched across the study districts, locating the chiefdoms and villages MCH aide trainers would be coming from. Judith's dog, Scamp, bit at my ankles, trying to interest me in play.

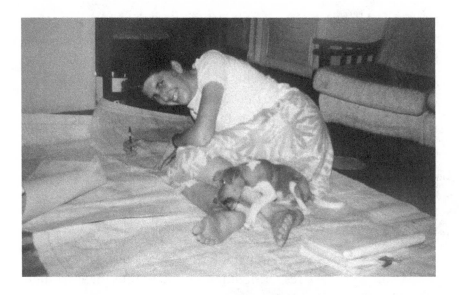

Identifying study villages on large government maps for research examining effectiveness of TBA training programs. Judith's dog, Scamp is trying to engage me in play (Bo, 1983).

Using a compass, I first drew a circle with a radius of three miles around each village with a health centre that was sending an MCH aide to the workshop. I then drew a line running north-south through each circle, and flipped a coin to determine whether villages on the east or west side of the line within the circle would be offered TBA training. The other set of villages were assigned to the control group. Their TBAs would not receive training. I listed control and study villages on foolscap, double checking the spelling of village names and making sure I had the right seven-digit enumeration area number for every study village.

I expected the workshop to be the more interesting part of the study process. I was thrilled to be Sister Fofana's training side-kick. I had seen her in action. I knew she could enthuse the MCH aides about their new TBA training role. She did not disappoint.

Sister Fofana and I taught using a mix of English and Krio. We introduced the reason for engaging MCH aides in TBA training, reviewed the content of TBA lessons, and shared adult education strategies. Half of the MCH aides indicated they had previously advised TBAs, often only one or two, concerning clean deliveries and preventing newborn tetanus. They all claimed to have met granny midwives in their area, but in most instances, only those who resided in the villages where they were posted.

We encouraged MCH aides to express their hesitancy about recruiting and training granny midwives. They explained the messy business of competing with granny midwives for deliveries and payment. This was a source of tension. Some believed TBAs threatened MCH aides' prestige as midwives.

Despite misgivings, the training conversation started to shift ever so slightly. MCH aides were beginning to consider how to reshape their relationships with granny midwives. They knew TBA training would add new work responsibilities. Five days into the workshop, they voiced tentative optimism regarding TBA outreach and training.

A lighter-side to the workshop was planned. MCH aides prepared teaching aids, sewing simple, newborn-size rag dolls, which they stuffed with Styrofoam. Scraggly bits of fabric were used to fashion umbilical cords. Cloth placentas were attached. We purchased large gourds in the market, one for every aide. The vendor cut a single hole in the centre of each calabash, giving each pseudo-pelvis a birth opening. The aides were now equipped with a set of demonstration teaching tools. MCH aides strapped the finished dolls on their backs, giggling as they pranced and sang TBA training lyrics.

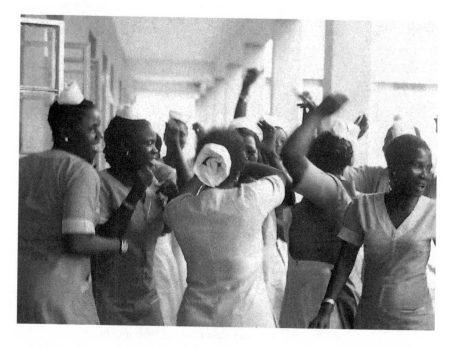

MCH aides practising TBA training songs during workshop in Bo (May 1983).

Defining moments of the workshop were about to come. Eight TBAs from several nearby villages were invited to join the MCH aides to *hang heads* and share their midwifery experiences. We sat in the cooling shade of a long veranda outside the training classroom. MCH aides wore their small white caps and faded pink uniforms. TBAs wore headscarves and colourful *lappas*. Their strikingly different attire set them apart.

I felt trepidation as we launched into a make-it or break-it exercise. Sisters Fofana and Samai began, inviting the granny midwives to describe how they became TBAs and to share their midwifery experiences. They did not hesitate, emphasizing their vivid stories with gestures and demonstrations. TBAs described how they conducted normal and complicated deliveries, how they knew when a baby was ready to come, and how they stimulated newborns to take their first breath.

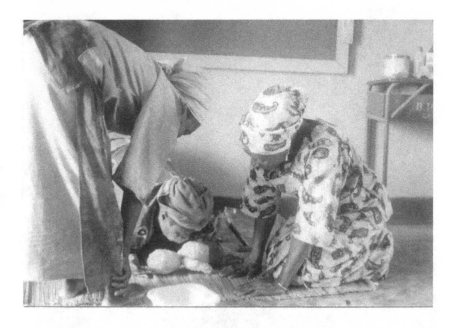

TBAs demonstrating how they stimulate a newborn to breathe.
The Styrofoam-stuffed demonstration doll was sewn by one of the MCH
aides during the training workshop in Bo (May 1983).

TBAs shared emotional journeys of good and bad delivery outcomes. MCH aides listened intently as the grannies spoke their truths. Despite the TBAs' lack of formal training, any bystander would have been impressed by their midwifery know-how. The mutual respect that existed between these granny midwives and villagers oozed.

The MCH aides pressed TBAs for more information about complicated deliveries. The TBAs' vignettes had sparked points of connection with the MCH aides—not only the joy of delivering a healthy newborn, but also the fear that welled up when labour stalled, when a newborn struggled to breath, when a woman bled heavily.

We then reversed the process. MCH aides described why they had enrolled as auxiliary midwives and what they had learned, first as students and then as practising midwives. MCH aides explained that they had started their midwifery work when they were young and before they became mothers themselves. Using stories of women whose births they had attended, the aides described clinical techniques for normal and complicated deliveries, explained which mothers they referred to hospital and why, and shared the angst of difficult referrals.

The sisters asked the TBAs to respond. I waited expectantly. The TBAs looked serious and earnest. One by one, they confirmed that they now realized these youthful MCH aides had *strong hearts*. This was the attribute *Bundu* Society *Sowey* deemed requisite for a woman to take up the TBA work. The granny midwives found the MCH aides to be bona fide in their skills and character. The TBAs thought they could acquire new techniques from the MCH aides to deal with the complications they feared the most, like postpartum bleeding.

My Mende whisper translator couldn't keep up with the rapid dialogue that followed this mutual sharing. Something momentous was underway. A double-barrelled change in perspectives was taking shape. The TBAs and MCH aides had started off on different footings, representing oppositional camps of midwifery practice. They were beginning to understand, appreciate, and regard each other anew. Their sharing had cinched a fresh beginning.

The warm glow of a mission accomplished replaced the apprehension I had sensed when we began the training exercise. Both groups of midwives wanted better outcomes for mothers and newborns. TBAs and MCH aides could work together on this common purpose.

Sister Fofana and I were confident that what had happened in the protective classroom setting would be replicated in the villages where MCH aides were to train traditional midwives. We had found a new starting point for MCH aide trainers—*hanging heads*. This was the Mende way for them to launch respectful dialogue with TBAs.

A few days later, my post-workshop euphoria started to lift. I was convinced that the MCH aide trainees would approach their work with TBAs differently. I thought our training had made a long-lasting difference. Yet, sorting out how to complete the TBA research study hung over me like a dark cloud. I was scheduled to leave the country in a few weeks. In brief, private moments of sober reflection, my research brain asked if the MCH aide workshop had been all for naught. I would have to return to Sierra Leone to complete the follow-up interviews in study villages. But how?

Staying On

I was on edge. I had been a persona-non-grata volunteer with the Bo-Pujehun project. This was not tenable for the long term. If I was going to return to Sierra Leone to collect follow-up data for my TBA study and complete analysis of the Bo-Pujehun baseline data, an alternate work arrangement was needed.

I broached a long, over-due discussion with Sister Hilary concerning my predicament. I explained that I wanted to continue my involvement with the Bo-Pujehun project and complete the TBA study. With my fellowship coming to an end, I could no longer do the baseline work as a volunteer. She agreed.

I left our meeting sensing a solution would be found. Sister Hilary indicated that the wheels had been set in motion for the project to employ me as an evaluator. Ministry approval was required.

Baseline data collection for Bo was complete. I had done preliminary data cleaning and analysis, tallying responses to questions in columns. Neat clusters of five strokes filled my work pages. Each hash mark represented a live birth or stillbirth, a maternal death, a neonatal tetanus death, an under-five child who was still alive, or a fully-immunized child. The ratios of positive to negative outcomes were not unexpected but distressing, nonetheless.

I presented some preliminary baseline results to Bo's District Government Health Committee. Findings were well-received. To my surprise, a committee member put forward a suggestion that they write to Sister Hilary requesting I be employed by the Bo-Pujehun project to continue work on the baseline data. This impromptu motion was supported unanimously. The endorsement was a nice pat on the back. It did not change my job status.

Sister Hilary had to address an immediate pragmatic matter. The EDCU assistants I had trained were still doing interviews in Pujehun District. She had drafted a letter for me to review in which she asked her counterpart, Dr. Komba Kono, to take over the Bo-Pujehun baseline study. My stomach turned as I read the letter. Given my temporary volunteer status, this transfer of responsibilities was an obvious necessity. I was reticent to let go. I wanted to be involved with the next steps of analysis and report writing.

Sister Hilary negotiated a new position for me with GTZ and Ministry of Health officials. Two weeks before my departure, a job offer came through. I was asked to return as a locally contracted employee with the Health and Nutrition Program of the Bo-Pujehun project to begin work after my planned leave in Canada. The new job would allow me to complete the TBA study, while gaining valuable work experience. I could put off my tangled inner debate about what long-term career path I was meant to follow.

I signed the contract for my new job as a monitoring and evaluation officer a week before my scheduled departure for Canada. With a surprising stroke of government efficiency, I got my residency visa renewed. I planned to return to Sierra Leone in August 1983. I now had a source of income for a fifth year in the country. It looked like I'd complete the TBA study.

I hired Sim, an EDCU assistant, and Agnus, an SECHN graduate from Serabu Hospital, to do reconnaissance work with the newly trained MCH aides in June and July. They were to assess progress, encourage TBA training efforts, and garner support from local Chiefs for the MCH aides to train TBAs. Sim and Agnus would maintain momentum for the hybrid arm of my study while I was away.

CHAPTER 27

BRIEF INTERLUDE AND FINAL YEAR IN SIERRA LEONE

My CIDA fellowship funding ended in June 1983. I headed back to Canada at the end of May with plans to return to Sierra Leone in August. My family was starting to wonder if I'd ever resettle in Canada to live and work. I didn't know myself.

As if life wasn't complicated enough, summer fanned the flames of love. I started dating a professor I had met while in graduate school. With this new passion in my life, it was going to be harder than I had expected to return to Sierra Leone.

My long-term career options were still a black hole of uncertainty. Summer brought unexpected employment opportunities. Following a chance encounter with colleagues at a conference, I was hired as a short-term evaluation consultant for a community health representative training program among First Nation's communities in Northern Ontario. This took me to several fly-in communities in Sioux Lookout Zone, where I got another taste of remote health care. I was reminded of health disparities between Ontario's urban and remote settings. There was important public health work needing attention in Canada, to which I might turn my attention if and when I came back to work in my country.

The innovative Northern program trained lay Indigenous community health workers from Cree communities. I was struck by commonalities between the Northern Ontario setting and Sierra Leone. The commitment of lay health workers and the regard their communities held for them exemplified principles of primary health care.

I applied for a temporary, part-time position with a new initiative, the McMaster-Aga Khan-CIDA Project.[28] [29] This entailed summer work in McMaster's School of Nursing and six weeks in Karachi that fall, teaching community health to baccalaureate nursing students. The Bo-Pujehun project Director agreed that I could take leave from my new position in Sierra Leone for the work in Pakistan. Although I felt like I might have taken on too much and was allowing myself to be pulled in too many directions, the short-term stint in Pakistan gave me a chance to augment my international development experience. This proved fortuitous as it led to a full-time faculty position at McMaster University after my fifth year in Sierra Leone. My career was sorting itself out.

Monitoring and Evaluation Officer

I returned to Bo in late summer, 1983. I had a spacious office in the one-storey, corn-yellow government building. A land-rover graveyard, filled with irreparable, broken-down vehicles, was within view. A human resource summary prepared for the provincial Ministry of Health indicated that the number of drivers and assistant drivers on government salary far exceeded the number of working vehicles. Too many funding agencies had budgeted for capital but not maintenance costs of vehicles. The heaps of non-functional vehicles were a constant reminder of the transportation malfunctions and broken referral systems in the Southern Province.

Work overload displaced my home sickness. I'd left Nick, my new beau, in Hamilton. We planned for him to join me in Sierra Leone for a few weeks in 1984 to get a taste of what life was like in my second home. I looked forward to Nick's visit and bridging his life experiences to mine.

Paul Sengeh joined me as my monitoring and evaluation counterpart. Paul had taught math and science in secondary school. He was a whiz with numbers and a fast-learner. Paul was a feisty, enthusiastic, and reliable co-worker.

Our work priorities were ambitious. Baseline data collection had been completed in Pujehun District while I was away. Computer entry and analysis of all baseline data could begin. I planned to finish writing the baseline study report. Paul and I would assist with the evaluation of primary health care training workshops that were getting underway. We set up a functional office and provided input on a review of the Ministry's information and reporting system. We designed and launched other health surveys. I welcomed the new sense of legitimacy I had with a formal position. Paul would take over my role when I returned to Canada in June 1984.

TBA Follow-up Interviews

I had permission to conduct the follow-up interviews for my TBA study alongside my monitoring and evaluation responsibilities. I got a boost when I obtained funds from the Commonwealth Foundation to partially cover fieldwork costs.

I debriefed with Sim and Agnus, who had visited MCH aides doing TBA training during my absence. I planned to start follow-up data collection for the TBA study a few months later. Interviewers would begin in Moyamba District, working in all villages that had sent TBAs to the government training. Follow-up data collection in Bo and Pujehun Districts would be completed in 1984. This gave MCH aide trainers about eight months to train TBAs. Still, timelines for the TBA follow-up data collection were tight. I tried not to fret.

Direct Field Supervision

In Moyamba District, I directly supervised assistants collecting follow-up data and saw their work challenges up-close. I relied on local transportation. My aim was to spend time with each of the seven enumerators assigned to this district on at least one occasion. I got to a third of the sampled villages, getting a small taste of the EDCU assistants' fieldwork.

Most of my supervisory contacts were brief. I located the enumerator who was already in the village and had a pro forma meeting with the Town or Village Chief. The interviewer and I reviewed completed questionnaires, discussed any concerns, and visited a few households. I worried that enumerators likened my efforts to scant supervision. This was not the case. EDCU assistants were pleasantly surprised when I showed up.

Escorts were provided when I walked from village to village. The burden of my travel fell on those who accompanied me.

Journal Entry

November 1983

Moyamba District

I walk back to the junction to catch a *poda-poda*, accompanied by two scrawny school kids who carry my bags. Oh, how I wish I had not packed so much. The children skillfully balance my bags on their heads, uttering not a word of complaint. On reaching the junction, we sit on a veranda eating *groundnuts* and bananas, while rehydrating ourselves.

A lot of transport goes past without even slowing down. The *poda-podas* are stuffed with people and goods. I finally get a lift to Moyamba, then on to Korgbotima. The EDCU assistant in this village welcomes me with a big smile. The assistant and I visit the Section Chief, the TBAs, and a few household members who have already been interviewed. Questionnaires have been filled correctly. The assistant looks pleased when I congratulate him on his work.

The assistant and I are given rice and *plassauce*. I head back to Moyamba by foot. At this time of the afternoon, traffic is exclusively one way, in the other direction. I'm accompanied to Pelewahun, a village two miles down the road, by the EDCU assistant and two secondary school children. They double back to Korgbotima. I continue on to Moyamba. I'm quite sure that if I stop moving forward, for even a moment, that will be the place I spend the night. My lodging comes into sight.

Encounters

Half of the sampled villages in Moyamba District were not motor-able. I travelled with EDCU assistants to less accessible villages, like Moyolo. Getting there involved a ride in an open lorry, a dugout canoe paddle across a narrow estuary, and an eight-mile walk. It was one of the few times I saw a snake on a bush-path. A green mamba, the length of a hockey stick, slithered across the path immediately in front of me. I came to an abrupt halt. My legs trembled. I tried to swallow my fear. I could barely whisper. My colleagues put their arms around my shoulders and comforted me, explaining that the snake was probably more afraid than I. There was a quiver in their voices. I moved to the middle of our walking line.

Half a mile from the village, we met the government-trained TBA, who happened to be my namesake, on her farm. She was pleased to see us and led us to her village where she introduced us to the Chief. TBA Nancy took Agnus and me aside to describe her midwifery work.

Journal Entry

November 1983

Moyolo

> The village of Moyola is small, yet there are five granny midwives. Only Nancy has been trained. She has done very few deliveries. A maternal death from eclampsia and a newborn's death prompted the Section Chief to send a TBA for the government training. He selected Nancy, his sister.

> I get a grand tour of the village including the *Bundu* hut. It is a dilapidated, mud-wall structure located at one end of the community. It has very little going for it with the exception of a zinc pan roof and being near enough to the river that TBAs have easy access to water during deliveries. I ask to see the inside of the hut. Reluctantly, one of the older grannies opens the creaky door.

The sudden stench of bat poop is unmistakable. Gingerly poking my head in, I'm greeted by at least ten bats circling the room. I'm too tall to stand up in the entrance way. I duck before timidly entering the dark, airless room. Two beds in the meagre hut are topped with straw. The filthy floor is thick with bat droppings. I cringe. The trained TBA assures me in Krio that the floor is swept before deliveries. I'm not surprised the grannies were hesitant to show me the room. Given the bat infestation problem, I suspect they are doing the deliveries elsewhere.

This was one of the worst critter problems I'd seen in a *Bundu* hut. The infestation suggested a lack of support from the Chief for the TBAs' work. While I had been meticulous in wording survey items, I had not asked enumerators to describe the condition of delivery rooms or huts. Completed questionnaires lacked any description of the reality-jarring, tell-tale contexts for village deliveries. That was an oversight I'd never forget.

The Royal Chair in Mokele

Mokele was one of the larger study villages in Moyamba District and difficult to reach. We'd be there for three days. I had the same trepidation I always sensed when heading off for an overnight stay in a village. Whose home would I sleep in, what kind of bed would I be offered, and would there be mosquito netting? What would be the state of village latrines? What nighttime creatures might I suffer?

Mokele means Black River; the village had been named for its location on the Telia. The river was bulging and fast-flowing; it looked dark and mean. Our team was shown to a roughly hewn canoe. One by one, we took off our sandals, stepped in the log, and quickly crouched to perch on narrow slats. We were all trying to tame the canoe's wobbles.

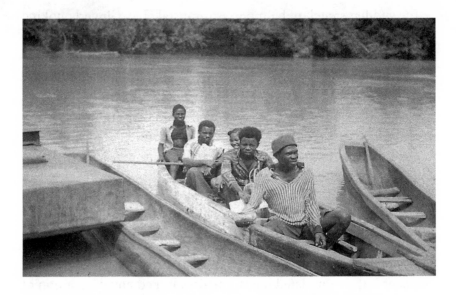

Dugout canoe travel. SECHN students positioned in middle;
boatmen sitting in bow and stern.

My feet were covered in water. Was there a leak? I saw no gourd or tin can for bailing. The boatman pushed us away from shore. I wasn't the only one clenching both sides of the canoe. My fingertips dipped into the river with each of the oarsman's paddle strokes.

The Town Chief and Chiefdom Speaker met us on the river bank and escorted us to the Paramount Chief, where we exchanged polite greetings. My attention was drawn to the Speaker's unique chair. A crown and QER II were carved into its upper segment. It dated back to the visit of Queen Elizabeth II in 1961, the year of Sierra Leone's independence. The chair was high-backed, like a throne. Had the Queen sat on this chair? And if so, where? Surely, she had not been escorted here via dugout canoe.

My momentary royal distraction was interrupted by the Paramount Chief explaining that he recently returned to Mokele. He had left the village months back due to a Chiefdom dispute involving accusations of corruption. The Chief was an educated man who had worked as a security guard at the mines before being elected Chief. He and the dispenser, who appeared intoxicated, started a round of verbal combat. The Chief barely kept his cool while the dispenser lashed out at him, claiming he had not been informed of our arrival until that morning.

The Chief ranted and raved about the unacceptable way the dispenser talked to him. He kept referring to section five in the National Assembly regulations that he could use to have the dispenser suspended. The Chief described himself as "head of state", saying he needed to discuss this matter in a cabinet meeting.

Data collection went well, despite the tension and rippling expressions of discord. At the end of our first day, we sat with the TBA to inquire of her recent government training. She explained that granny midwives in the area were afraid to go to a place as distant as Moyamba for training. She believed other TBAs might be willing to travel to the next training since they had seen her come back with new midwifery skills.

At dusk, I was shown to a highly irregular bathing site: a wooden box where I was invited to sit. The box had been placed under a large shade tree, 200 or so feet from the Chief and other villagers who were debating where I would be lodged. A bucket of tepid water was brought to me by a school-age child. I washed my face, neck, and extremities; I was not going to reveal any other grungy body parts to onlookers. The traditional, enclosed wash yard surrounded by palm fronds was situated within sight of the wash box. I was not invited to use it until the second evening. *How for do.*

The next day, the Chief addressed a group of TBAs from nearby villages who had walked to Mokele. He asked the Speaker to read aloud my letter about our visit and to then translate it to Mende. The Chief launched into a lengthy monologue regarding the price of rice and other commodities. His entire harangue was in English. No Mende translation was offered. The grannies shifted on their stools but remained respectfully expressionless.

Despite the Chief's strange introduction, I was confident the trained TBA would impart useful information to the traditional midwives who had taken the time to come. She was a social influencer, a trainer in her own right. I left the TBAs talking while I joined household interviews. We finished our survey work late in the afternoon.

At daybreak, the dispenser grabbed his paddle, briskly rounded up our team, and escorted us to a canoe for the return trip. I supposed the Paramount Chief and his nemesis were relieved to see us go; they had a palaver to settle.

Early light flickered through the haze of small cooking fires; a shimmer danced on the river. My receding view suggested a peaceful village. I admired the dispenser's doggedness. His day-to-day work involved navigating the temperament of a cranky Chief.

I was thankful for the dialogue we'd had with the TBA; she seemed a peace-maker. The study questionnaires were capturing only a smidgen of the vital work TBAs undertook in their villages.

I looked forward to sleeping in a familiar bed, protected by mosquito netting. My sense of humour kicked back in. With a parting glance of Mokele, I considered writing a letter to Her Majesty, inquiring about the throne.

Indirect Field Supervision

As we had done for the baseline survey, government supervisors were assigned to the EDCU assistants collecting TBA study data in Bo and Pujehun Districts. I provided indirect supervision, debriefing enumerators when they returned to Bo. Their feedback gave me a glimpse of their village work.

I paid overnight allowances and reimbursed transport costs for EDCU assistants. When enumerators returned to Bo, they were in need of a break, and past ready to spend time at home. They just wanted me to attend to administrative matters. As one of my journal entry affirms, sometimes I missed their cues.

Journal Entry

February 10th, 1984

Bo

Thirteen EDCU assistants have returned from the villages after collecting data for the TBA study. I spend the morning with them along with their field supervisors going over problems that arose. Their main complaints are notification of Chiefs, and feeding and lodging. In Galu, they claim not to have been fed for several days.

Three assistants who worked on the Sumbuya side of the Chiefdom tell me they had sore muscles from walking to the villages and went to the dispenser looking for an injection. Two were given procaine penicillin and the third streptomycin. They were told to return for two more doses of antibiotics. I am keen to discuss this matter at length [as I consider this to be an occupational health and safety issue]. It's a teachable moment concerning the dangers of misusing antibiotics.

The assistants must think I'm daft—they only want to collect their transport allowance. At last, I get down to the payment business.

I gleaned information from enumerators' written reports. One interviewer indicated that when he arrived in more isolated villages, women ran away with their children because they were afraid of hut taxation business. In other villages, TBAs thought enumerators were coming after them because they'd refused to go for government training. Field reports gave me pause. No matter how well intentioned, interviewers could add to the angst of women and TBAs living in study villages. Other than re-explaining purposes of the study and making sure proper consent procedures were followed (villages and households had the right to refuse interviews), I had no suggestions for EDCU assistants on these unfortunate matters.

CHAPTER 28
A BLOOMING RELATIONSHIP

I knew that stepping into Sierra Leone was going to be a shock for my boyfriend. Nick had never been to that part of the world. Flexibility was not his strong point. I was anxious to show him around. His visit, which was part work and part vacation, would be a reality check on whether we should seek deployment as a couple for a work term in a less-developed country. I had filled him in on some of my experiences as a CUSO volunteer. As his arrival neared, I upped the details through letters and audio-tapes.

We were in for four intense weeks with highs and lows, emotionally and figuratively. Our relationship deepened, but new fissures opened up between us. Traversing our experiential divide was complicated.

Because of the McMaster University connection to Fourah Bay College, Nick planned to run a few epidemiology tutorials for district-level government employees. Teaching was his strong suit. Nick communicated difficult methodological concepts with ease. His well-attended sessions were held in a provincial Ministry of Health office. He made me proud.

Nick caught me up on current Canadian and international news. For the first few days, I welcomed this information because my sources of global news were so spotty. I had enjoyed updates when I was back in Canada. Now that Nick was in Sierra Leone, I tired of this conversational focus. Global affairs seemed irrelevant to my day-to-day life and work. I was detached from international happenings and lacked the mental energy to absorb them. Rather than offering us a point of common interest, they generated a sense of disconnect.

Being an amateur astronomer, Nick was taken with the more southern sky. Blackouts in Bo made for good viewing on clear nights. Holding me in his arms, he tutored me in cosmic formations. I cherished our closeness as we star-gazed.

When it came to food, Nick was cautious; too cautious, bordering on picky. I accommodated some of his food preferences, although I was determined to expand his repertoire and delighted when he tried local dishes. It annoyed me when he insisted that we spend time one Sunday afternoon going to the small shops in my neighbourhood in search of 7 Up, his favourite soft drink.

I got my come-uppance in a village where we had been invited to a celebration. We were among the honoured guests taking in drumming and dancing ceremonies under the blazing sun. A traditional meal was offered, starting with chili pepper soup. A Krio explanation about the dish was provided by the young dancer who handed us soup bowls. I understood what she said; Nick did not. Before I had a chance to translate, Nick had uncharacteristically gulped down a big spoonful of the fiery hot liquid. His face turned red like the peppers he'd swallowed. He was gasping, desperate for a drink. But there was no potable water, nothing to alleviate the burning that engulfed him. He remembered little of the ceremonies that followed.

Nick accompanied me to several peripheral health units. I wanted him to see health care in the villages. For me, getting to and from these locations was a routine part of the work. For Nick, travel was disquieting and frightening. After one particularly long day at a health centre, we began our ride back to Bo in a project vehicle. The driver navigated the rutted and rocky track. We lurched in our seats. By the time we reached the main road, the evening was pitch black. Lorry drivers turned on their headlights as we approached them on the narrow, two-lane highway. Blinding high beams leaped out of the darkness like foreboding monster eyes. Intermittent headlight use was supposed to save battery life; but it created hazardous night-driving conditions.

Nick was nearly apoplectic, grabbing for my arm with each passing vehicle. I judged he was over-imagining the travel risks. His risk-averse reactions brought my questionable, fatalistic-coping attitude into view. My dismissive efforts to reassure him fell short.

At the end of Nick's visit, we enjoyed what for me was an extravagant two-night stay at a hotel overlooking Lumley Beach. It was a romantic and playful setting that tamed my workaholic tendencies and gave us time to reflect on the weeks we had just spent together. We frolicked in the ocean waves, strolled on the soft-sand beach, and enjoyed dinner and dancing at a shore-side Lebanese restaurant. À la carte breakfasts were served on a small patio, surrounded by fluorescent pink and orange blooms of hibiscus and bougainvillea. We had a gorgeous vista of the glistening Atlantic that linked and divided Canada and Sierra Leone.

My usual accommodation in Freetown was the austere, but safe, women's hostel run alongside a school by religious Sisters. I was used to the sparse dorm room with its creaky wood floor, where guests slept on narrow, iron-spring cots with thin mattresses. Our short stay in the Lumley Beach Hotel was palatial in comparison. Never before had I felt like a tourist in Sierra Leone. I much preferred my sense of belonging as a resident worker.

Seeing Nick off at the airport was tough. While we had differences, we were falling in love and had enjoyed moments of tenderness and affection in my adopted African home. Although Nick had found the adjustment to Sierra Leone difficult, I knew he had been taken by the nature of my work, the dedication and talent of my Sierra Leonean and international colleagues, and the challenges health workers overcame. We had both realized that if our relationship progressed, working as a couple for extended periods of time in a less-developed country was not in our cards.

I accompanied Nick to the airport where he had to navigate one last challenge. He was carrying a few locally made baskets. The airport authorities demanded that he pay a tax for his "antiquities". That absurd request translated to *an ask* for a bribe. Using my best Krio, I objected. The request was withdrawn. Nick was waved through customs with his woven souvenirs that still held the scent of grass. He was unhappy to leave me, but eager to head home to more familiar territory. I was abruptly pulled back to the realities of my fulfilling work in Bo.

CHAPTER 29
BITTERSWEET

I was up against another deadline; this one was bittersweet. The end of my fifth year in Sierra Leone neared. Work was running on impossibly tight timelines. Completing analysis of the baseline study had turned into an insurmountable pre-departure challenge. Power sources and computers were not cooperating. The analytical work would have to be completed once I got back to Canada.

One Apple II computer had been allotted to Bo's project office. Early in 1984, when Paul and I were partway through the baseline data-entry escapade, the computer broke down. It was sent to West Germany, the closest repair shop. We waited impatiently for a German colleague who finally returned with the computer just as Bo-wide electrical power outages got worse. The power was off for days at a time; the backlog of computer work piled up. Paul and I weren't the only staff waiting in line with data to be entered or analyzed. We completed baseline data entry.

I had booked my airline ticket home. My full-time faculty position at McMaster would start in July. I aimed to draft a preliminary report of results before I left. The tight deadline left me weak in the knees. My ensuing insomnia proved timely. I was joined by Mark, the project's computer geek, to run frequency checks and begin descriptive analysis. This took all-nighters—the only time we could get a turn on the computer. We relied on a portable generator that ran on diesel. It powered a lightbulb and the computer. Crowing roosters signalled daylight when we'd free up the computer for others.

I submitted the preliminary baseline report a few days before leaving. Findings would guide health and nutrition program directions, and provide comparative indicators for a later round of data collection to assess project impact. I brought the data home on floppy disks for further analysis and with plans to write a more detailed report. New headaches would stall the next phase of analysis.

Paul and I put the completed baseline questionnaires in green garbage bags and locked them in the wooden cupboards of the Bo-Pujehun project office. As far as I know, nobody ever looked at them again. During interviews, families had shared their raw emotions about live births, stillbirths, and deaths of women and children. Responses had been recorded in tick boxes, with a few words of explanation sometimes entered in the margins. Each event had been converted to a single, data-entry keystroke and then anonymously summed and buried in the calculation of health status indicators. Locking the questionnaires in dark cupboards metaphorically silenced the fulsome stories of hope and joy; of sorrow and tragedy.

The health indicators were inert, bare-boned numbers, bereft of human-story backdrops. My epidemiology training had equipped me with quantitative analysis skills. I was aggrieved by the countless, lost stories behind the numbers. Although I recognized the power of numbers, gut punches came from stories. If I was going to use research to make a difference, I needed to augment both my quantitative and qualitative research skills.

Heading Home

TBA data were still coming in from the villages a few weeks before I was due to leave. None had been entered on the Apple II computer. I planned to carry completed TBA questionnaires back to Canada; there were no feasible alternatives. Judith and I stuffed the reams of paper into my canvas knapsack, trying not to rip the pages as we used up the last slivers of space. The knapsack barely closed. I worried the weight of my backpack might tear the leather shoulder straps.

On departure day, I jostled amongst a determined group of elbow pushers at the airline check-in counter, praying I would not be asked to put the knapsack on the foreboding scales. It would put me over the weight limit. I could be charged a hefty fee and worse, forced to check the knapsack as baggage. The mental image of my data-filled bag disappearing into the global abyss of lost luggage made my heart pound. I took deep calming breaths.

Sweat dripped down my torso and legs. The leather straps gouged, my back ached. As I approached the counter, I stood up straighter to make it look like my chockablock backpack was lightweight. The ticket stuck to my moist palms as I handed it over and uttered a chatty Krio greeting. *"Morning oh. How di body?"* I don't think my deceitful behaviour fooled the airline clerk, but she gave me a break. She didn't weigh the knapsack, and she didn't query its hand-luggage status. I breathed audible sighs of relief as I found my seat on the plane and placed the precious cargo between my feet. I wasn't going to let the questionnaires out of my sight.

The enormity of the moment gripped me. My sense of relief shifted to a feeling of chaotic disruption. This journey back to Canada marked a turning point in my life. Would I lose hold of the unfaltering global health and development direction that had been my guide? I was excited to return to Hamilton to rejoin my boyfriend and to begin my faculty position. Serendipity was surely at play, but was it leading me in the right direction?

I was overcome by nagging questions I had put aside in the flurry of intense work. When and how would I return to this country, whose people I loved? Could I make a meaningful contribution to international development from an academic position in Canada? Was leaving Sierra Leone a bad decision, a choice I would regret?

I turned my head and pressed my forehead against the window. Tears rolled down my cheeks, a gravelly lump lodged in my throat. Images flashed through my mind—nursing students, traditional midwives, Chiefs, Serabu's public health team and religious Sisters, and government colleagues. I was going to miss the work. Most of all, I would miss the people. Nothing could replace the friendship, comradery, kindness, courage, and life lessons they had shared. I would not forget the heart-warming and heart-breaking stories of families and birth attendants.

Although the mountains of Freetown would soon slip from my sight, memories of Sierra Leone and its people lay deep within me.

Part 5
Back in Canada

"Yesterday, I was clever, so I wanted to change the world. Today, I am wise, so I am changing myself." (Rumi)

CHAPTER 30
UNFINISHED BUSINESS

I started my faculty position in the Nursing Department at McMaster University in July 1984. I'd have to squeeze analysis and report writing for the TBA study and baseline survey into my faculty workload. It felt daunting but doable. The urgency of this unfinished work was being replaced by new academic demands on my time. Had I been completing the research in Bo, my Sierra Leone colleagues would have pressed me for updates and aided my interpretation of study findings. They had a stake in the results. I missed their day-to-day comradery.

I was working with data from two studies. I felt strongest ownership of the TBA data. Some of it had been coded. Data entry was the next step. I purchased a portable computer, the weight and shape of a loaded, medium-size suitcase. Its six-inch black screen had lime-green lettering that strained my eyes. I had intended to use my new computer to enter and analyze all of the TBA data but reverted to hand-tallying some results.

The Bo-Pujehun baseline data was on floppy disks. There was no going back to the questionnaires if errors surfaced. I'd have to analyze this larger data set on a main-frame computer in McMaster's health sciences computing facility.

TBA Research Results

The research design for the TBA study was a tad complicated with three sets of study villages. I had randomly assigned eligible villages in Bo and Pujehun Districts to either hybrid training or control groups. Study villages in Moyamba District had received the government training. I hypothesized that villages in both TBA training groups would have better outcomes than those in the control group.

In total, there were 82 villages in the MCH aide hybrid training group, 68 in the control group, and 21 in the Moyamba training group. Response rates were high. Chiefs had permitted interviews in 95%, 93%, and 100% of hybrid, control, and Moyamba study villages, respectively. Follow-up interviews had been conducted with all practising TBAs and all mothers of child-bearing age who resided in the three sets of villages.

Most TBAs in the study villages were farmers (>85%), over 40 years of age (80%), and had no formal education (>95%). In comparison with TBAs trained in Moyamba, TBAs in villages assigned to MCH aide training were more often head TBAs (44% versus 32.7%), practising herbalists (14.6% versus 11.8%), and learned midwifery skills from a relative or friend (27% versus 19.1%).

Hybrid training

All 20 MCH aides had made headway with TBA training in their assigned villages in the eight months since they'd completed the workshop in Bo. However, MCH aides reported delays. Some had waited to start training until TBAs' farm work lightened. One MCH aide was preoccupied with additional responsibilities because the dispenser's position in her health centre was vacant. In a couple of villages, tensions between health workers disrupted training efforts; an unqualified woman posing as a nurse-midwife in one community, and a village maternity assistant who was competing with TBAs for deliveries in another.

Chiefs expressed support for TBA training, although some were slow to mobilize the participation of TBAs in study villages. One MCH aide was befuddled when enthusiastic TBAs from control villages asked to join her training. The unambiguous list of intervention and control villages on my master sampling sheet belied complex relationships that cut across study villages.

MCH aides' records of TBA attendance were a bit spotty. The number of granny midwives that each MCH aide reached ranged from three to ten, and these TBAs had attended approximately 80% of the MCH aides' training sessions. Nine days of training for 20 MCH aides had yielded over 100 trained TBAs in less than a year—a good multiplier effect.

Knowledge, attitudes, and practices

TBAs were individually asked knowledge, attitude, and practice questions about prenatal, labour and delivery, and postnatal periods. How can newborn tetanus be prevented? How do you examine a pregnant woman? TBAs residing in study villages assigned to the hybrid training out-performed TBAs in control villages, while Moyamba-trained TBAs did not. Specifically, TBAs in the hybrid program most frequently reported checking pregnant women for anemia and swollen limbs, and palpating the abdomen, and they were the most knowledgeable about ways to prevent tetanus, though their scores weren't perfect.

I had set a higher bar for health outcomes than the government evaluation of trained TBAs. All TBAs in study villages were interviewed, whether or not they had been trained. This meant that scores for the granny(ies) who had been trained were combined with scores for untrained TBAs in the same village. This approach likely lowered the average TBA score assigned to a village but it was consistent with the pattern of who did deliveries post-training. Untrained TBAs in Moyamba's study villages were still in the delivery-business. They had conducted nearly half (46%) of the TBA-attended deliveries in their villages after the Moyamba workshop.

Group practices

Since TBAs often worked together to conduct deliveries, their group practice was also assessed. Using a prepared checklist, interviewers asked TBAs in each study village to assemble and jointly demonstrate a set of clinical skills. To mimic a real delivery, they invited a pregnant woman into the hut normally used for deliveries.

TBAs in the hybrid program had significantly better scores for history-taking, hand-washing, physical assessment, and delivery room and equipment preparation than TBAs in either Moyamba District or the control group.

Other indicators

Tetanus immunizations and antenatal clinic attendance rates were lowest for villages in Moyamba District, and higher for both hybrid and control villages. Women in hybrid training villages reported twice as many deliveries in a health centre and by an MCH aide than women in either control or Moyamba villages. This was a promising result in the hybrid villages although we could not ascertain the risk status of mothers who were and were not delivered by personnel with more training than TBAs.

Interviewers had recorded plenty of births (542, 399, and 281 births in hybrid, control, and Moyamba's villages, respectively). There had been 24 neonatal deaths in total; a neonatal mortality rate of 19.6 per 1,000; over 40 times higher than Canada's rate of 0.41 per 1,000.

Differences in neonatal mortality between either set of intervention and control villages were not statistically significant. Neonatal mortality rates were slightly lower in the hybrid villages (16.9 per 1,000) than in either control (17.7 per 1,000) or Moyamba villages (25.2 per 1,000).

Across the three sets of villages, neonatal tetanus had caused 41.6% of all neonatal deaths; 22.2%, 37.5%, and 71.4% in hybrid, control, and Moyamba villages, respectively.

Although results in the hybrid training looked clinically promising, they were not statistically significant. Statistically, the sample size of 171 villages and 1,222 births had fallen short.

Neonatal tetanus deaths were still taking place, even after TBAs had been trained. These results reinforced the importance of tetanus toxoid immunizations for all women of child-bearing age. TBAs could encourage women to get immunized but a reliable and functional immunization program had to be in place for this messaging to work.

The hybrid approach had reached and trained more TBAs faster and at a lower cost to the Ministry than the centralized government training in Moyamba. A longer period of follow-up was needed to determine if improvements in knowledge, attitudes, and practices would last.

There had been insufficient time between training and follow-up to adequately assess neonatal mortality outcomes. I hadn't expected either TBA training approach to reduce maternal mortality given intransigent bottle-necks in the obstetrical referral system. Training TBAs alone was not sufficient to ease structural barriers.

Reporting the results

A year after leaving Sierra Leone, I sent a preliminary report of results about the hybrid training to my research funder, the Commonwealth Foundation. I published a couple of articles describing the work of TBAs in Sierra Leone[30] and shared preliminary findings at several conferences. In 1988, I presented the main results at an international conference.

I didn't think the knowledge, attitudes, and practices results were publishable. These had been reported in other studies of TBA training. The primary outcome I had pegged as novel was whether or not TBA training led to a reduction in neonatal mortality outcomes including newborn tetanus. Those results were not conclusive.

For a couple of years after I left Sierra Leone, I held out hope for another round of follow-up interviews to assess neonatal mortality rates. That opportunity never came.

I have two main regrets. I did not send a report of study results to Dr. Williams, and I did not publish the main results. I put off writing a report for the CMO, thinking that soon enough I'd have a peer-reviewed publication to share with her. I attempted to publish results in a post-conference book chapter following the international conference presentation. I sent a draft to the editors, who indicated the manuscript needed more work. I was not able to meet their publication deadline.

I set my sights on publishing in a journal but then concluded that the negative neonatal mortality results were of little interest. That was a lame excuse. I started full-time PhD studies in 1988 and diverted my attention away from writing-up TBA study findings. Results slid into the realm of too-long-since-study-completion to be publishable.

I should have written up results of the hybrid training as a proof-of-concept and invited contributors to that training program as co-authors. We had increased the coverage pace of TBA training by preparing auxiliary midwives as trainers.

Many individuals had propelled the study forward. Without Sister Hilary's credibility and support, my study plans would have ground to a halt at the permission-granting table. Serendipity had played out in favour of launching the TBA study and completing data collection. Sister Hilary's new position in Bo, her invitation for me to assist with the Bo-Pujehun baseline survey, and the offer of a contractual position for my fifth year in the country had all been fortuitous stepping stones. The tenacity of interviewers who endured formidable field conditions, the talent of nurse Fofana who led MCH aide training, the enthusiasm of the auxiliary midwives to train TBAs, and the willingness of households to disclose personal information had all made the study possible. I let all of them down by not sending a report of, or publishing, the main study results.

The TBA study had not yielded the breakthrough reduction in neonatal mortality rates I had hoped for. I had experienced firsthand the incremental nature of science. I had seen the limitations of a follow-up period that was too short to properly assess the impact of TBA training on mortality outcomes. The hybrid training had not tackled systemic barriers to maternal or neonatal health care.

Nevertheless, a vexing health care delivery problem—how to scale-up TBA training in a setting with enormous health human-resource constraints—had sparked a novel research question and an innovation in TBA training. Research ideas could unleash viable approaches for primary health care delivery. Research was a tool for change.

Bo-Pujehun Baseline Analysis and Results

With more powerful computers at McMaster, I supposed that further analysis of the baseline data would be straightforward. It proved stubbornly difficult.

Nick offered the computer programming assistance needed to transfer data from floppy disks to a mainframe computing system. That task exceeded my skill level. He faced numerous complications and incompatibilities. Who would have guessed we'd be hampered by computer problems at McMaster?

We eventually located an Apple computer that we could freely access. It failed to read data from the floppy disks I had brought back to Canada. We needed a copy of the technical manual for the Apple II computer we had used in Bo to sort out the incompatibility challenge. Nick and I retrieved that information on a return trip to Sierra Leone in 1985. It had taken nine months to navigate a few technical difficulties.

The not-so-simple matter of efficiently transferring data followed. We completed transfer to the Apple computer in August 1985. Next came data transfer to McMaster's mainframe computer. Fortran code had to be written so the format would take up less computing space; we had squatter's rights on the mainframe. Again, I relied on Nick's generosity to write the program language. By the time data were ready for analysis, I was weighted down with teaching responsibilities. I completed analysis on weekends. On and off, I wrote the report.

Sister Hilary waited. On February 1, 1986, she sent me a letter, stating that a consultant from the German government was soon arriving to review the Bo-Pujehun project. Ongoing financing of the initiative (from June 1987 onwards) would be determined during his visit. She was quite sure he'd ask for the baseline results and implored me to send the long-overdue report. That was the kick-in-the butt I needed to finish the work. I was terribly embarrassed. I had not met my promise to deliver a timely final report.

Key findings

I started off the report with the conventional numerical summary of villages surveyed. The final tally showed we had data from 294 villages in Bo District and 235 villages in Pujehun District. Given the field difficulties enumerators had faced, the high response rate was a notable accomplishment. In Bo District, data was collected in 88.8% of the sampled villages. They had reached over 95% of the estimated population in participating villages. Interviewers were refused permission to work in five communities. Thirty-three villages were deserted.

The response rate in Pujehun District was lower. The survey was completed in 75.6% of the sampled villages. Fifteen villages were deserted. In 61 villages, enumerators were refused permission or unable to complete the work, largely due to political unrest. The instability had been wider spread than EDCU assistants' field reports indicated. Enumerators had reached 80.2% of the estimated population in Pujehun's study villages.

As expected, basic infrastructure was lacking in both districts. Most study villages (88.2% in Bo, 87.4% in Pujehun) had no schools and no adult literacy classes. The proportion of villages with all-weather, four-wheel drive motorable roads was 49.4% in Pujehun and 37.4% in Bo.

Over 50% of households used rivers, streams, or swamps as their primary water source. Less than half had access to a latrine. Safer drinking water sources (protected wells, spring boxes, and pipe-born water) were used by a mere 8.6% and 8.4% of sampled households in Bo and Pujehun Districts, respectively.

Families reported deliveries, maternal deaths, and the survival or death of under-five children in the year prior to the survey. EDCU assistants had obtained information on 1,372 deliveries (live and stillbirths) in Bo, and 1,201 deliveries in Pujehun. Over 87% of women who had given birth had no formal education.

The majority of births (71.2% in Bo and 83.2% in Pujehun) had been attended by untrained TBAs, usually in a home or *Bundu* hut in the pregnant women's villages of residence. MCH aides had attended 6.7% of births in the two districts. The TBA training coverage rate problem was abundantly clear. Only 4.5% of deliveries had been attended by government-trained TBAs, and 1% by Mission Hospital-trained TBAs.

Physicians had attended a mere 0.4% of reported deliveries. The caesarian section rate for the two districts was an astoundingly low 0.13%. One third of all deliveries attended by physicians were for mothers requiring caesarian sections. Most women requiring a caesarian section had never made it to the hospital or arrived too late. Their numbers were buried in maternal mortality, stillbirth, and neonatal mortality rates.

Maternal mortality rates were mind-numbing: 444 per 100,000 in Bo District, and 422 per 100,000 in Pujehun District. These numbers were 25 times higher than the maternal mortality rate in Canada.

The challenges of accessing hospital services partly explained high maternal mortality rates and the low number of hospital deliveries. On average, households in both districts had to use two modes of transportation to get to the nearest hospital. The average cost for motorized transport to a hospital for one person, one way, was Le 5.40 in Bo and Le 12.76 in Pujehun;[31] these amounts were more than the average monthly income of most farming households.

Infant mortality rates (proportion of babies who died under one year of age) were 91 per 1,000 in Bo and 127 per 1,000 in Pujehun, more than ten times the same rate in Canada. Mortality rates for children under-five years of age were 143 per 1,000 in Bo and 165 per 1,000 in Pujehun. Commonest causes of children's deaths were newborn tetanus, measles, and gastroenteritis. These three conditions accounted for 37.4% of all under-five deaths in Bo; 53.9% of all under-five deaths in Pujehun.

Enumerators had collected data on thousands of children under-five years of age: 3,534 in Bo and 3,163 in Pujehun. Nearly half (46.1%) of the children in Bo had an under-five card compared to

23.7% in Pujehun. Immunization rates in Pujehun District seriously lagged.

I wasn't surprised by the appalling health indicators, which confirmed what we had found in the villages of Bumpe Chiefdom during community assessments. The statistics were mothers, newborns, young children, and families. The harsh mortality figures left me with a penetrating sense of sorrow. Precious lives lost, way too soon.

Feedback on the baseline report

I didn't ask and never heard if the baseline results directly factored into the German Government's decision to continue funding the Bo-Pujehun Rural Development Project. I received two letters regarding my report. One was encouraging, and the other discouraging.

Sister Hilary informed me that my report had been given to the GTZ consultant evaluators. They were pleased with it. Baseline data on water sources informed a large village water supply program funded by the State-owned German Bank.

Dr. Griffith, a community health physician with the Bo-Pujehun project was based in Pujehun. He wrote me a discouraging letter. He didn't want my report to sit on a shelf. He diplomatically alluded to the delay in getting my report, noting that in the two years since the baseline data had been collected, transportation costs from a peripheral health unit to the government hospitals had increased nearly ten-fold. Referral bottlenecks were getting worse.

Then he got to the crux of the matter. Some results in my report had been questioned. Infant and under-five mortality rates were lower than those that had been calculated indirectly using 1974 census data, by a well-known demographer at Njala University College. In his letter, Dr. Griffith stated: "The baseline figures had been rejected by the Ministry of Health in Freetown." The biggest discrepancy was for Pujehun District: infant mortality census data estimates were 294 per 1,000, while the report's baseline rate was 127 per 1,000. He asked if I could think of any reasons for the discrepancies.

The only explanations I offered were the sample of study villages (a large proportion being within three miles of a peripheral health unit) and the 24% village refusal rate in Pujehun District. Possibly, excluded villages had higher infant mortality rates than included villages. I maintained that the lower infant and under-five mortality rates in Bo District were plausible given better immunization rates. I too was concerned that our estimates of Pujehun District's mortality rates were lower than expected.

Maternal mortality rates for Bo and Pujehun Districts were high. They had not budged in a decade. Ministry officials had not questioned those figures.

CHAPTER 31
RE-ENTRY AND RECALIBRATION

My return to Canada in June 1984 was permanent. I was positioned uncomfortably on the other side of the poverty gulf. I found the adjustment difficult. Simple, day-to-day activities in Hamilton held constant reminders of life in the villages where I'd worked.

I was overwhelmed by the abundance of food in grocery stores. I felt incapable of making a selection. I longed for a market with limited choices, where my cash went right into the hands of a vendor who was eking out a living.

I found food waste repugnant in restaurants, food courts, and at home. Waste was a potent reminder of difficult hungry seasons. I'd remember little ones with kwashiorkor or marasmus being so lethargic they neither played nor ate.

Hearing water running from a tap was nearly intolerable. I'd immediately be taken back to images of women and children carrying buckets of non-potable water to their homes.

When I saw kids playing during school recess, I squirmed with the thought of mothers cobbling together enough cash to pay for their youngsters' primary school fees and uniforms. An educational trajectory for village children that involved post-secondary school education was unimaginable for most small-scale farmers.

Sometimes, I was overcome with emotion during special celebrations and overwhelmed by the injustice of disparities that registered in my psyche.

Slowly, upsetting flash-points came to mind less. My attention was absorbed and distracted by new circumstances, new relationships, and new expectations.

Re-Entry

During my years in Sierra Leone, I had grown and matured. I came back changed. My metamorphosis was hard to explain. I wanted to share experiences so that family and close friends could better understand what had reshaped me. But sharing left me emotionally raw, and I became less and less inclined to do so. Most people were interested in brief anecdotes, maybe one or two. The humankind connections I hoped to channel through stories too often went awry. Interest was whetted by their exotic elements, not by their raw messages.

My stories were understood and treated as travel stories. Superficially annoying questions or comments followed. When a probing question was asked, I found it challenging to provide an adequate response. How could I embed my answer in a description of the broader socio-cultural context? Did communicating what I had learned from the Mende people abuse my privileged outsider status?

I was certain that my experiences in Sierra Leone were applicable and instructive for public health in Canada. My attempts to draw parallels were misconstrued. Colleagues argued that primary health care in low-income countries was second- or third-rate health care. I found these views narrow-minded and frustrating. Slowly, I got better at describing pertinent public health examples from Sierra Leone so they were not dismissed immediately.

I eased back into Canadian life. I thought less about disparities between Sierra Leone and Canada and more about disparities close to home. Inequalities between homeless and housed, between Indigenous and settler populations, and between citizens and refugees started to grab my attention.

In the spring of 1985, I returned to Sierra Leone to teach a three-week epidemiology course for West African diploma students enrolled in the Community Health Program at Fourah Bay College. Nick, who by then was my fiancé, taught a biostatistics course over the same period. It was good to be back in my second home. I was surprised yet relieved that my yearning to return for a longer stay in Sierra Leone had lessened. I was preoccupied with planning my wedding. I was settling into my new life in Canada.

Recalibration

The political situation in Sierra Leone was deteriorating. Conditions for conducting field research had become increasingly precarious. In 1986, Sister Hilary sent me a letter describing the worsening situation.

> We had no fuel last week. For the first time I saw the lorry parks without a single vehicle. You can't believe it. *Pan top*, the new government slashed all prices, whereupon the vendors carried their goods. Home? Nearby villages? God knows where. But there was NO food in the market last week. We were all caught without supplies ... there are general elections in May, and one hopes they will be "free and fair". But nobody should be out in the villages in the middle of an election campaign.

I reread the letter, absorbing her message. My involvement in any ongoing research in Sierra Leone had ended. My heart sank. There would be no return trips for another round of the Bo-Pujehun baseline survey. Additional research in the villages where TBAs had been trained was out of the question. Whether or not government-trained or MCH aide-trained TBAs reduced neonatal mortality rates in the long term would remain unanswered questions.

Sister Hilary had hinted at much worse political instability that was yet to come. March 1985 had marked my last pre-civil war visit to the country.

The letter was a career wake-up call. While political unrest terminated the possibility of further research in Sierra Leone, other doubts had been settling in my sub-conscience. Sierra Leoneans with extensive public health experience, some with graduate degrees, were fully capable of doing the evaluation work. Paul Sengeh had completed his master's degree in statistics at McMaster. He had taken up a permanent position with the Bo-Pujehun project and was in charge of the monitoring and evaluation portfolio. My skills had become redundant.

In principle, I knew this was the desirable outcome of international development work. But I had a sense of disquiet. My pre-existing work ties to Sierra Leone had been permanently disabled. I was re-questioning my future role in international development.

My aspirations for a career with a global health research focus seemed increasingly remote and unrealistic. After returning from our short trip to Sierra Leone in 1985, Nick and I had prepared an application to evaluate a retraining program for peripheral health unit staff in Bo and Pujehun Districts. We submitted the proposal for funding to IDRC. It was turned down. Canada's main global research funding agency was focused on building research capacity in lower-income countries; their funds were directed to the nationals of those countries. Given IDRC's mandate, rightly so. However, without funding sources, I figured my global health research days might be over.

I got involved in global health development initiatives at McMaster University. I mentored international students connected with the McMaster-Aga Khan-CIDA Project. I organized overseas clinical placements for medical and nursing students. I tutored in a community health training program offered by the African Medical and Research Education Foundation in Kenya, and joined a short World Health Organization-led workshop on TB in the Philippines. I participated in a mid-term evaluation of the McMaster-Aga Khan-CIDA Project. These international activities were satisfying sidelines.

However, I struggled to sort out the direction for my academic research. Public health matters in Canada did not peak my interests in the way so many health issues in Sierra Leone had. How would I ever land on a research topic as pressing as preventing newborn tetanus or maternal mortality, or scaling-up TBA training?

In 1986, I took on a joint appointment with the public health department in Hamilton. The new role provided an inroad for me to network with managers and staff in the local public health unit. I got my research funding feet wet with a health promotion project involving immigrants and refugees living in Hamilton. This was a swing-bridge to my interests in global development. Yet, I still missed being directly involved in all phases of research in a low-income country. Nothing matched the excitement of such purposeful inquiry.

Reconciling Life and Career Goals

On the home front, I navigated life and career goals. I was married and hoped to have children. If I wanted to continue in an academic position, I needed to get my PhD. These goals were complicated enough without factoring in my global health research aspirations.

I knew my husband could not settle happily into a long-term stay in a third-world country. I had met international couples who had thrived in Sierra Leone; others had found it difficult. I had seen relationships fraught because one of the partners found living and working overseas unbearable.

The prospect of children raised other concerns. While living in Bo, the German nutritionist who worked with me on the Bo-Pujehun project had lost his toddler to an acute gastrointestinal infection. The little one's tragic death left a heavy burden of guilt. If I had children, I didn't think I could bear such risks.

I had talked to British colleagues working in Sierra Leone who had teenagers. Their children were enrolled in boarding schools back in England. Parental visits were limited to holidays. Such forced separations were not what I wanted for my offspring.

I still pined to be involved in international development work. Paradoxically, the inequities that had drawn me to this quest, pushed me away when it came to my family. Canada would be my home base for any future global health career opportunities.

CHAPTER 32
A REBOOT

Four years after returning from Sierra Leone, I found myself in the midst of major life events. I put my brief sojourns of international work on hold. My husband and I moved to eastern Ontario, where Nick started a new faculty position at the University of Ottawa. I commenced PhD studies at McGill and took on part-time teaching and local public health consulting in Ottawa.

My son, Andrew, was born in 1989. My life was full as I balanced motherhood, PhD studies, and work. Then, a bombshell hit. In 1990, I was diagnosed with cancer. Months of treatment followed. I focused on being a mum and getting well. I came close to quitting my PhD studies.

The ground wobbled. I felt vacant of purpose on the global health research front. Other than my involvement as a board member with the Canadian Society for International Health, I was in the midst of a four-year hiatus from international development work. I occasionally yearned to spend time in West Africa, but in 1991, Sierra Leone's civil war began. That country's door was shut tight.

I still hoped that a new opportunity for global health research in a low-income country would emerge. Failed efforts to get IDRC research funding for a study in Sierra Leone had left me stymied. My PhD thesis topic addressed maternal and child health among immigrants and refugees living in Ottawa. These women's stories kept my global health research light lit.

Another Continent

The School of Nursing at the University of Ottawa, where I started a full-time faculty position in 1992, had no collaborative projects with African institutions. However, several faculty were involved in a nursing education initiative in Tianjin, China that was funded through World University Services of Canada. It was one of the Canada-China University Linkage Projects initiated following the Tiananmen Square incident of student-led protests in Beijing in 1989. The Canadian Project Director was leaving for another position. Shortly after beginning my faculty appointment, I was asked to take on this role. I would need to make short trips to China, once or twice a year—travel I could balance with family responsibilities.

I was a People's Republic of China newbie. My Chinese counterpart, Madame Zou Dao Hui, Director of the Nursing School of Tianjin Medical University, provided outstanding leadership, co-guiding project implementation.

Tianjin Medical University is in China's third largest municipality—an industrial, coastal metropolis. Two aspects of this capacity-development initiative were of particular interest: mentoring junior faculty to do research, and integrating community health content in the curriculum. I had moved back into the international development arena, albeit not on the continent (Africa) where I wanted to work, not with a primary focus in public health, and not with a mandate or budget to do research. Nevertheless, capacity development was a worthy objective.[32] [33]

I was committed to the work in Tianjin although I missed the challenges of close-up, public health work in rural and remote communities. When an opportunity to get involved in a bilateral project in Yunnan Province, People's Republic of China came along, I enthusiastically agreed. My PhD was done, my son was school age, and I was healthy.

I reasoned that the Yunnan project was a chance to renew and revive my evaluation and research interests in rural primary health care. Feasibility had already been ascertained. I soaked in details of the proposed project from briefing materials. The health statistics for Yunnan's rural counties read like those of a third-world country. I was invigorated by the possibilities of this work.

In 1996, enlivened and nervous, I embarked as the Canadian lead for the design mission of the Yunnan Maternal and Child Health Project. Several other Canadian experts joined the mission, notably Susan Smith, who I had worked with on the McMaster-Aga Khan-CIDA Project. She was a participatory-training guru.

Dr. Zhan Wentao, Yunnan's Acting Deputy Director of Public Health, was the Chinese lead for the mission. He was a gregarious physician whose specialty was Traditional Chinese Medicine. He spoke a few words of English. He led a group of public health colleagues, who collectively had decades of experience in training, deploying, and supporting village doctors and village midwives. These cadres of health workers were still the backbone of Yunnan's primary health care delivery system. The deployment of barefoot doctors dated back to the Cultural Revolution. They offered primary health care in rural and remote villages; working within a referral matrix of township, county, and prefecture hospitals.

Our bilateral CIDA project was to be undertaken in ten ethnic-minority and poverty counties. Six of these counties were co-located in the western part of Yunnan, in and around Lijiang. At the time of our visit, several project counties were smack in the middle of a disaster zone. Buildings had crumbled and lives had been lost when a massive earthquake hit a few weeks previously.

International aid was pouring in. Clinical staff were still working out of temporary tent hospitals when we arrived. At first glance, it looked like modern buildings withstood the earthquake best. I was mistaken. The structure of some buildings had buckled. They were no longer safe for occupancy. Red tape blocked doorways. They would have to be demolished and rebuilt.

The brick walls of some traditional buildings had collapsed inwards, taking young lives. The toll could have been much worse. The massive wood frames for the much older, two- and three-storey buildings were still standing. The traditional framing structures were earthquake proof. They swayed rather than collapsed with the forces of a quake, saving lives and speeding up the rebuild. I was reminded that traditional knowledge and craftsmanship are important in all sectors.

Reaching Lijiang involved an 18-hour drive from provincial government headquarters in Kunming. Along with senior members of Yunnan's provincial Health Bureau, our Canadian group was cooped up in the multi-vehicle convoy for this journey. The long trip gave us plenty of discussion time that exhausted our translator. We delved into matters like how Western and traditional health care systems operated in tandem, what continuing education village doctors and midwives had received over their decades of work, and how to rapidly scale-up training. Dr. Zhan Wentao primed me on the autonomous governance structures of the ethnically-diverse project counties. He and his colleagues introduced me to some of the Indigenous peoples of Yunnan: Naxi, Bai, Lisu, Dai, and Yao.

On endless hairpin turns and undulating roads up and down mountainsides and through lush tropical valleys, Dr. Zhan and I got into the thick of experience-sharing. I dug into my Sierra Leonean primary health care stories, emphasizing community engagement strategies and participatory training. Dr. Zhan shared facts and anecdotes about Yunnan's village doctors and midwives. His team described the hierarchical, top-down, train-the-trainer approaches they had been using to reskill and upskill village, township, and country health workers with a World Bank loan. These senior staff were overseeing implementation of this cascade training in other Yunnan counties.

Our Chinese colleagues urged us to adopt a cookie-cutter version of the World Bank train-the-trainer model for the new CIDA project. This became a contentious point of debate. The distinctions Susan and I made between the more didactic training approaches they were already using and the participatory methods we were proposing were nuanced, and lost in translation. I tried putting forward supporting evidence for participatory primary health care, but it did not convince. I then used anecdotes of village health committee and TBA training in Sierra Leone to illustrate the strengths of bottom-up community involvement to propel health improvements. My West African anecdotes were the basis for a breakthrough in our disagreement. Dr. Zhan and I absorbed the thrill of a newly found aha moment.

Dozens of site visits to health care facilities and lengthy planning meetings followed. Participatory training and evaluation became core elements of the maternal and child health project. We jointly agreed on guiding principles, developed implementation details, and prepared the proposal for submission to CIDA. All project documents had to be translated from English to Mandarin. I realized we had co-created new approaches to the rural health work in Yunnan when our Canadian project team was told that no Chinese characters existed for several key English terms used in the project document.

I worked with a translator who used my explanations of key concepts to painstakingly construct Chinese characters that conveyed their notional meaning. We verified logograms with Yunnan colleagues. We were building a lexicon. I had never had to dig so deep to explain the meaning of public health terms that rolled way-too-quickly off my tongue. The concepts of community engagement, participatory approaches, and community dialogue took shape in Chinese character strokes. Translation processes had cut to the quick, untangling fundamentals of the Yunnan project for English- and Chinese-speaking team members.

What stood out for me in those early days of the Yunnan project was how my experiences in Sierra Leone resonated with my Chinese colleagues. More than a decade after I had left West Africa, Serabu's primary health care and TBA training programs provided a common touch-point for sharing on the other side of the globe.

CIDA and Yunnan's Health Bureau co-funded the ambitious maternal and child health project for nearly six years. CIDA provided $5.6 million in development aid.[34] I was excited to be co-leading a project that reached poor families in remote areas of southwest China. My counterpart, Dr. Du Kelin had assumed her position as Deputy Director of the Provincial Bureau. We had an excellent working relationship.

No research objectives and no research funds were attached to the project. To my dismay, CIDA had instructed me not to use the "R" (research) word in the application. We budgeted for an external evaluation using data from Yunnan's robust maternal and child health surveillance system. End-of-project results were encouraging, showing a 30% decline in maternal, neonatal, and infant mortality rates that exceeded a downward trend for these mortality rates in Yunnan Province.[35]

Canadian-Centric Research Program

Despite my enthusiasm for this international development project in Yunnan, I had pretty much given up my aspirations for global health research funding. By the end of the 1990s, my funded research projects and my organizational research partners were all in Canada. My research interests had expanded to include other public health issues like preventing falls among seniors and implementing best-practice guidelines for nurses.

My Canadian-centric research reality was cemented in place. In 2000, I was awarded a ten-year Nursing Chair from the Canadian Health Services Research Foundation. All the research I described in my application was Canadian-based. The Foundation had stated clearly that research in low-income countries was not eligible.

Eleven other colleagues were awarded Chairs in the same national competition. I was perplexed and upset to learn that other awardees had international research activities planned, albeit in higher-income countries. I debated this discrepancy with the Executive Director of the Foundation several times. He did not budge.

I was mired in the same old quarrel predicated on opinions that health services research undertaken in less-developed countries had little or no relevance for Canada's health care system.

I must be head-strong. I ignored the remit envelope of my Chair award when I co-applied for global health research funds that became available a couple of years later. The proposal, which tackled environmental tobacco smoke in China, was funded. In my annual

Chair report for the Foundation, I tucked the description of that research into my portfolio of development work in China.

Global Health Research Funding

In 2001, the Canadian Institutes of Health Research was established. The mandate of this major health research funder included global health services research. Canadian academics were eligible to apply. The funding landscape had started to change, just when I had a program of research fully situated in Canada.

More changes on the funding landscape were afoot. Several Canadian agencies forged a new partnership in global health research, and with this came larger-scale funding opportunities. The Foundation had done an interim evaluation of my progress as a Chair and approved continuation of my award for the full ten-year period.

I still wanted to venture back into global health services research. I figured the Foundation had given up trying to keep me on the straight and narrow course of doing health services research in Canada. My rebellious tendencies surfaced.

One of my post-doctoral trainee fellows, Judy Mill, had invited me to join a health services research initiative on HIV and AIDS that she was leading in Canada. Her project provided a jumping-off point for us to develop a multi-country program of research to build the capacity of front-line nurses and nurse managers to improve the quality of care for persons living with HIV and AIDS. Researchers from four low- and middle-income countries (Jamaica, Uganda, Kenya, and South Africa) joined the team along with researchers from several Canadian universities.[36][37] I co-led the work with Drs. Dan Kaseje (Great Lakes University of Kisumu, Kenya) and Eulalia Kahwa (University of the West Indies Mona, Jamaica). My involvement in other funded international projects followed, including research led by Dan to examine the scale-up of a maternal and child health initiative in nomadic and agrarian areas of Kenya.[38]

With these funded global health services research projects, I had bridged the career divide of research in Canada and in lower-income countries—and I was back working on the African continent. The Canadian Health Services Research Foundation had either given up on my global health research forays, or come around. They were no longer questioning the relevance of my global health research activities, at least not in my presence. By 2007, I was profiling my global health research projects alongside Canadian studies in my annual Chair reports.

An Opportunity

I got one more kick at the global health research can when, in 2008, I took the helm as Scientific Director for the Institute of Population and Public Health with the Canadian Institutes of Health Research.[39] My predecessor, Dr. John Frank, had been the scientific lead for global health research. He was one of the instigators of the multi-agency global health research partnership with IDRC, Health Canada, and CIDA.

Work undertaken through this partnership was the forerunner of a maternal and child health initiative in Sub-Saharan Africa that came partially under my watch. A multi-country, Global Health Research Alliance in Chronic Disease Prevention was also getting its footing. I was part of these multi-agency efforts, steering an implementation science agenda with other funders. Multi-million-dollar investments in research funding aimed to reduce inequities by tackling structural determinants and improving the coverage and scale-up of effective interventions. All Canadian researchers funded through these global health initiatives were required to work with principal investigators in partnered countries. Translating knowledge to action was a major thrust of these health services and population health research programs.

My career had come full-circle. I was on the funding end of the research chain, stipulating application requirements that were intended to attract some of the world's best scientists to address intractable health services delivery problems. I was still reaching back to my days in Sierra Leone as a source of inspiration and ideas. While I had a stronger and more diverse set of international experiences to draw on, those from Sierra Leone were the rock-solid, foundational illustrations I repeatedly turned to.

A Final Thanks

Over the years, I have delved into my Sierra Leonean encounters, sensed their unsettling forces, and applied them to other work opportunities and life circumstances.

I remain abundantly thankful to the generous people of Sierra Leone who shaped my views, values, and spirit. The powerful village stories and human truths imparted to me reverberate within. I have mental images and emotional flashbacks that are as vivid for me today as they were when I lived in the country. These experiences continue to fuel my drive for human betterment, for a more equitable world.

A framed photo of Mansaray with her four children in the small village of Blama has sat on my bureau for over three decades. I see her family's portrait when I awaken each day. Mansaray reminds me that all of humankind have the power of advocacy for progressive change. She is one of my permanent inner voices, and to her I say with gratitude. "Yes, Mansaray, I left Sierra Leone, but Sierra Leone never left me."

CHAPTER 33
PERSONAL REFLECTIONS

Through the passage of time, I've come to terms with two disquieting aspects of my Sierra Leonean experiences. I once considered these topics off-limits to divulge or discuss. Their emotional overlays run deep.

Female Circumcision

I skirted the topic of female circumcision when I was in Sierra Leone. This practice was not a health priority for Serabu's primary health care program. It seemed intrusive to probe for information about the practice, and audacious to provide commentary on Secret Society initiation rites.

The term "female genital mutilation" (FGM) was adopted by the World Health Organization in 1991.[40] What followed was an extraordinary turn-around in global attention for a practice I had not even heard of before I arrived in Serabu. I have watched the growing international movement for FGM eradication from the sidelines. My regard for TBAs in Sierra Leone leaves me conflicted.

The words female genital mutilation/cutting (FGM/C) are both evocative and provocative. My Western leanings urge me to think that FGM/C, as practised among the Mende, is a symptom of disempowerment; of women being forced to undergo a procedure that demeans and harms their bodies; a violation of human rights. FGM/C suggests that men have the upper sexual hand, and girls have no choice when there should be consent. You might expect me to be a vocal critic of FGM/C. But that's not the position I've taken on this matter because, among the Mende, female circumcision is a ritual of the *Bundu* Society.[41] [42]

I hold that long-lasting and progressive change is more likely when social institutions are respectfully engaged. That's why we were so excited when Serabu's TBAs decided to make tetanus toxoid immunization part of the *Bundu* initiation ceremonies.

I'm not a *Bundu* member. Therein lies the rub. Insights about how the *Bundu* Society offers protections for girls and women, alongside its circumcision practices, are largely out of my reach. I think it's too cavalier to simply strike down what outsiders label a culturally-offensive practice. Such a stance risks threatening or dismantling safeguards offered by cultural institutions, such as strict *Bundu* Society laws that forbid voyeurism and incest.

Some prominent female advocates such as Fuambai Sia Ahmadu have argued that the term FGM/C represents a Western intrusion of powerful and degrading language intended to turn Mende girls and women against a revered Mende institution.[43] Some Sierra Leonean women who are pro-FGM/C have argued that well-respected members of the Society would be tainted by bans on circumcision. The organization *Sierra Leone Women are Free to Choose*, launched in 2016, was an offshoot of this thinking.

Recognizing the power and strengths of the *Bundu* Society,[44] the government of Sierra Leone has worked more closely with *Bundu* leaders over the last decade. The legal substrate for a shift in FGM/C in Sierra Leone was enacted in 2007. This is when the Child Rights' Act was passed; children are defined as those under 18 years of age. The Act offers stronger and more definitive legal protection for children in the country. Passage of this Act was spurred on by horrors of Sierra Leone's civil war and, in particular, youth who were forced to become child soldiers.

Sierra Leone's National Gender Strategic Plan 2010-2013 followed,[45] and the 2013 Agenda for Prosperity included a pillar on gender and development.[46] The 2013 Agenda called for a ban on girls under the age of 18 being put through the Secret Society's rite of passage (circumcision).

Government recognized that the *Bundu* institution needed to co-lead this social change process. On May 19, 2017, *Sowey* converged in Waterloo, on the outskirts of Freetown. They affirmed their willingness to uphold the government's decree to ban female circumcision among children if parliamentarians continued to show their respect for the authority of the *Bundu* Society. Their stated position was clear.

> Many of the *Sowey* from across Sierra Leone, personally thanked the Honourable Minister of Social Welfare, Gender and Children's Affairs—Dr. Sylvia Olayinka Blyden for sticking out her neck in protecting and promoting women of the *Bundu* Society to exercise their constitutional right to associate together across the country. The *Sowey* repeatedly assured the Minister that they would follow the policy to the letter and convince fellow women to do likewise, whilst also undertaking self-policing.[47]

Efforts to stop FGM/C in Sierra Leone have brought other matters to light. *Sowey* have identified the need for financial protection from government since initiations that do not include circumcision lower their earnings. In a country with no universal social security net this is a big issue. Shifting the practice of FGM/C has repercussions that must be understood and attended to. Changing a cultural rite is one thing; retaining the long-standing strengths of gender-specific social institutions is quite another. The *Bundu* Society, its *Sowey*, members, and initiates are rewriting their own history. TBAs are leading the way for a pivotal change to the practice of FGM/C in Sierra Leone. Momentous change comes from within.

I am still troubled with the question of an appropriate role for me, a public health nurse, a Western woman, and a cultural outsider in relation to female circumcision in Sierra Leone. A partial answer came to me during a chance rendezvous in Dublin in 2019. At the time, I was visiting Sister Hilary. She introduced me to an Irish priest who was working with an international organization to prepare a report on the causes and devastating health consequences of vesico-vaginal fistulas, which affect several million women, almost entirely in low-income countries. He asked me if and how this condition was related to FGM/C. I was taken aback because I had never asked this question of myself, not even while supervising a post-doctoral fellow whose PhD thesis had been on the topic of vesico-vaginal fistulas among Ghanaian women.

In response to the priest's question, I had a cursory look for reviews of evidence on the relationship between FGM/C and fistulas. In one of the few published population-based studies using demographic and health surveys from more than 25 Sub-Saharan African countries, FGM/C was not a direct risk factor for vesico-vaginal fistula. However, lack of education, defined as not being able to read, increased the odds of an obstetrical fistula by 13%.[48] I had a long-overdue realization. Lack of education for women tops the list of risk factors for maternal deaths. The same structural cause had multiple, devastating health outcomes.

Education is a powerful intervention because it informs decision-making. It engages, it bolsters, and it provides the basis for a wider set of choices. I had a partial answer to my FGM/C cultural-outsider dilemma. Advocating for better and more accessible formal education for children and for adult literacy classes for adults, principally girls and women, provides an alternate entry-point for change and health improvements by a cultural outsider.

Do I have regrets regarding my inaction on FGM/C while I was in Sierra Leone? My answer is "no and yes." Serabu's public health team had to pick its battles. We chose to work with TBAs and the *Bundu* Society to reduce newborn tetanus and maternal mortality. These were the communities' priorities: preventable causes of death that were the source of much angst and heartache. Early successes were likely. The practice of female circumcision met neither of these criteria. Taking on female circumcision would have undermined our relationships with TBAs and deterred progress on their expressed health concerns.

While much of my work in Sierra Leone involved training and education, I failed to grasp the profound importance of primary education. Young Fodia made frequent visits to my village home in Serabu; I never asked her mother about Fodia's schooling. During community assessments, we did not document whether or not school-age children were enrolled in primary or secondary schools. Our education information was too sparse to tally sex differences among school attendees and non-attendees. Such indicators would have been a jumping-off point to discuss children's access to Sierra Leone's formal educational system with the Chiefs and TBAs, an entrée to advocate for girls' primary and secondary education. I regret having not paid enough attention to the formal education of girls and women when I lived in Sierra Leone.

Sierra Leone's Civil War

It was 1995. The civil war had escalated. Rebels were encroaching on Serabu. The Sisters received word that armed security men at the mines had failed in their attempts to defend international workers from the rebels. No security staff were employed at Serabu Hospital. Any semblance of safety for the hospital's personnel vanished in a heartbeat. Sierra Leonean staff fled, fearing repercussions due to their hospital affiliation. The Sisters narrowly escaped to Freetown. Within weeks, there was an exodus of expatriates. I heard these descriptions from the Sisters years after the civil war ended.

In Canada, real-time news of Sierra Leone's civil war came in fits and starts through the media. I am ashamed to say that for the most part, I turned away from the war's horrors. Unease tormented me when I heard of atrocities and reflected on my passive inaction. I found news of the civil war distressing, sickening, and appalling. Reports got worse, and worse again. I could not imagine the terror that war was striking at the heart of Sierra Leoneans.

I was living another reality. Same planet but a different world. My son and his friends were thriving in the safety and security of peace in Canada, while a cohort of Sierra Leonean children were experiencing the destruction and disruptions of war merely an ocean away.

Teens had been ripped from their homes to become child soldiers. Each of these children, their families, and their villages had experienced unthinkable and inhumane brutalities. Reflecting on these horrors still makes me shudder and leaves my cheeks wet with tears.

Other than private conversations with colleagues who had worked in the country, I said next to nothing to either friends or family about the civil war. When I heard reports of the relentless brutality, a sense of guilt settled in my core. I was filled with reproach. I saw no way to provide any direct aid. I stood aloof. Years passed.

Although a peace accord was reached in July 1999,[49] the war was not declared over until January 18, 2002. The excuse of civil war that I held onto as a reason for not visiting the country evaporated. Thankfully, the war was no longer. I could safely return to Sierra Leone, see the situation for myself, and renew friendships. I hesitated, stalled, and dithered. Slowly, it came to me that I did not have the courage to go back, not to Serabu, and not to the country. I wanted to reminisce about Sierra Leone and the people as I knew them. Sierra Leoneans had been through unspeakable trauma. Family life, village life, and farm life had been turned upside down and literally slashed and burnt. People and communities had been torn apart and stamped out. The war must have seemed interminable.

I renewed efforts to connect with friends and colleagues from Sierra Leone. At the top of my list was Sister Hilary. We had kept in touch through correspondence, but I had not seen her since 1986. After leaving Sierra Leone, she was redeployed to Cameroon to set up another primary health care program. In 2000, she retired in Dublin.

I couldn't fathom how she came to terms with 42 years of working in Sierra Leone alongside the country's tragedy of war. In 1984, the President had awarded her the highest honour for an expatriate, Commander of the Order of Rokel. Sister Hilary had planned to retire in her beloved *Salone*. She had even looked into applying for citizenship. Instead, she was back in Dublin living in a community with other displaced and retired Sisters. Sister Hilary wrote of her experiences among the Mende. She became President of the

Sierra Leone-Ireland Partnership, successfully advocating for Sierra Leone to be designated a priority country for Irish development aid. Physically, she lived far away from Sierra Leone; mentally she was in its midst.

My visits with the Holy Rosary Sisters in Dublin were occasions for sombre reflections, alongside unfading journeys down memory lane. Several Sisters I had worked with in Serabu Hospital had left their religious order.

Some of the Sisters, including Mama Hilary, had been back to Sierra Leone for short trips. All spoke of the grief and sorrow they felt on their return. The brunt of the war's destructive forces had descended on Serabu. Early on, the hospital and convent were burnt to the ground by rebels. Mega-damage was inflicted on the compound. In photos, it looked like the hospital had been bombed.[50] During my last visit with Sister Hilary, she spoke again about this destruction. She was still trying to understand the unthinkable, to make sense of the senseless. What had fuelled this symbolic and wanton ruination of a hospital and its staff that had been Serabu's pride and glory? I had no answers. We uncomfortably closed that dark pit of inquiry.

I pressed international colleagues who worked in Sierra Leone after the war for information. I gleaned bits and pieces of news regarding former students and co-workers. Some had been internally-displaced. Others were back in the country after time spent in refugee camps, where they had waited for the war to end. My Sierra Leonean monitoring and evaluation counterpart (Paul Sengeh) and a colleague who had studied at McMaster (Dr. George Gage, Head of the Community Health Department, Fourah Bay College) were involved in post-war and post-Ebola rebuilding.[51] I sorrowed over news of Dr. Victor Cole's death. Victor was a stalwart champion for primary health care, having served as National Primary Health Care Coordinator and then the first Principal of Bo's Paramedical School. Dr. Williams had retired in England.[52] Each story triggered sober reflections.

By 2010, the country and its people were getting back on their feet. A long healing journey lay ahead. The health situation was improving, although HIV and AIDS had arrived and TB remained a big problem. The country was rebuilding its health service infrastructure, training and retraining health workers, and renewing its primary health care efforts.

In 2015, the Ebola crisis hit, bringing another humanitarian catastrophe, wreaking its havoc through more unspeakable trauma. Nearly 20% of the country's health care workforce died of Ebola.[53] Women stopped going to clinic. Schools closed. Primary health care services were decimated. Health care in the country went backwards.[54][55]

Sadness heaped upon sadness. I did not think I could bear to see the devastating consequences of the civil war or the after-math of the Ebola crisis. My knowledge of the situation in the country was going to remain secondhand. War and epidemics did not define Sierra Leoneans, but these tragedies had most certainly and unfairly shaped their lives.

I have never lived in a war-torn country. Doing so is unimaginable. Yet, I am acutely aware of the personal irony. Television images of Vietnamese children who suffered the atrocities of another senseless war in the 1960s had first sparked my desire to work overseas.

A Look Back

Much time has passed since I left Sierra Leone. Where does my slow-burn development leave me now, as I enter my retirement years and take on a new role as grandmother for my precious grandson, Oliver?

Now in my seventh decade, I am less naïve than my younger self. I've seen that public health improvements usually come in small increments. Along the way there are steps forward, backward, even sideways, and then forward again. The change process involves plenty of real-time adjustments and adaptations. My preferred timelines have nothing to do with the actual period required for transformation, nor do they define an optimal pace for this process.

With the advantage of hind-sight, I have advice for my younger self:

Take risks; serendipity will play a part.

Learn new truths by listening to others.

Dig deep through periods of difficulty.

Don't take yourself too seriously. You'll mess up from time to time.

Feel the depths of human connections. Let these rouse your compassion, your humour, your love, your outrage, and your determination to better the human condition.

Watch for your cultural blind spots. They can pop up unexpectedly. They are tempting to dismiss. Heed them.

Change takes tenacity and more time than you think you have. You may want to give up. Values reenergize. Mentors support.

The future rests on the shoulders of youth. I have beginning advice I hope to impart to my young grandson:

Even the smallest and quietest voices matter.

Join hands and lock arms to make things better.

It takes many sleeps to change big things.

Finale

In November 2019, I travelled to Dublin, where I visited Sister Hilary and three other Sisters I had worked with in Serabu. We had several days together. This was a joyous reunion, peppered with back-stories, humorous anecdotes, and conversations about our lives and work in Sierra Leone.

Sister Hilary and I reconnected instantaneously, like close family. We were tethered by memories that spontaneously welled up. I urged Sister Hilary to share her stories. I'd heard them before; they still brought fresh laughter. Most had an element of Sister Hilary's typical self-deprecation. "Remember when I bought a goat at the market? I bartered for a good price. The goat disappeared. Another Sister bought the same goat later that day. She too, got a good price."

Sister Hilary invited me to her small private room in the convent for cherished alone-time. We bantered. "Did I like the way she had rearranged her furniture to make it easier to get around with her walker? What did I think of the forthright instructions she'd given the support worker who provided her evening care? Was it reasonable for her to still have writing projects?"

We dove deep and shared confidences. Sister Hilary reflected on recent conversations she'd had with a priest about the meaning of life. I shared the emotional visits I had with my dad during his last months in long-term care.

We talked relationships: her niece Alice, my son Andrew and my ex-husband, Nick. We caught up on siblings. Most of hers long-gone; my younger brother and youngest sister now mature adults with families. We spoke fondly of our mothers, mine 94 years old and thriving, her mother who had passed.

We chuckled, remembering a religious slip 35 years prior. Her mother had blessed me with a small splash of holy water as we were leaving Sister Hilary's family home in County Mayo. When Sister Hilary reminded her ma that I was not Catholic, a generous handful of holy water swiftly dampened my clothes.

We discussed adversity and hope; inequities and development aid; Brexit and Trump. We chatted about getting older and being old; youthfulness and learning from younger people in our lives. Sister Hilary was full of life and optimism. We both thought Serabu Hospital's primary health care program had made a difference. We mourned the losses and tragedies of Sierra Leone's people.

In those moments of sharing, we reached back to our beloved *Salone*. Reminiscing and reconnecting with Mama Hilary felt sacrosanct. That was our last time together. Sister Hilary died peacefully in her sleep on January 11, 2020.

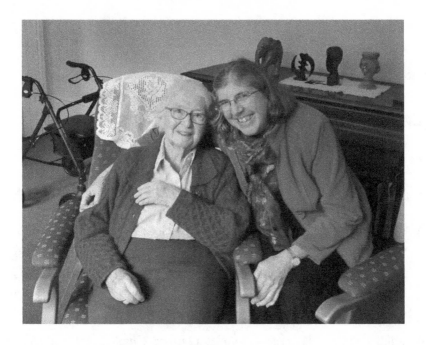

My final visit with Sister Hilary Lyons (Dublin, 2019).

Notes

Chapter 1: Arriving

1 Canadian University Services Overseas (CUSO) changed its name to Cuso International in 1981.

2 Ian Smillie, *The Land of Lost Content: A History of CUSO*, (Madison: Deneau, 1985).

3 Arrival of the 1,100 Nova Scotians in Freetown is detailed in Leo Spitzer, T*he Creoles of Sierra Leone: Their Responses to Colonialism 1870–1945*, (Ile-Ife, Nigeria: University of Ife Press, 1975), 10-12.

Chapter 2: Panoply of Health Services

4 Hilary Lyons, *Where Memories Gather: Chuckles and Wisdom* (Glasgow: Dudu Nsomba Publications, 2009), 37.

5 Hilary Lyons, *Letters to Alice*, (unpublished manuscript, 2018), 44.

6 Lyons, *Letters to Alice*, 52.

7 Lyons, *Letters to Alice*, 52-53.

8 Lyons, *Letters to Alice*, 46.

9 Lyons, *Letters to Alice*, 41.

10 Lyons, *Letters to Alice*, 59.

Chapter 5: Housing and Housemates

11 Ross Carey, *Notes of a Medical Student*, (Personal Correspondence, 1984), 8.

Chapter 9: Play, Learning, and Celebrations

12 Sylvia Ardyn Boone, *Radiance From the Waters: Ideals of Feminine Beauty in Mende Art*, (New Haven: Yale University Press, 1986).

13 For a detailed description and photos of Sowey masks, see: Boone, *Radiance From the Waters*, Chapter 5, Sowo: The Good Made Visible, 153-244.

14 For a detailed discussion of masks and masking, see: Ruth B. Phillips, "Masking in Mende Sande Society Initiation Rituals," *Africa* 48, no. 3 (1978): 265-277.

Chapter 11: Revamping Community Assessments

15 For a discussion of ancestral spirits and other Mende beliefs, see: W.T. Harris, and Harry Sawyerr, *The Springs of Mende Belief and Conduct: A Discussion of the Influence of the Belief in the Supernatural Among the Mende*. (Freetown: Sierra Leone University Press, 1968).

Chapter 12: Expect the Unexpected

16 For a description of the Serabu Hospital experience using drama see: Nancy Edwards, "The Role of Drama in Primary Health Care," *Educational Broadcasting International* 14, no. 2 (1981): 85–89.

Chapter 13: Poverty in the Raw

17 Nancy Edwards and Simeon Sisay, *Findings of the General Baseline Survey Health and Nutrition 1980/81*, Magbosi Evaluation Section Information Bulletin Series no. 2 (1981): 1-11.

Chapter 14: Witches

18 Primary Health Care in Bumpe Chiefdom Six-monthly Report: January 1981–June 1981 (1981), 9.

19 Primary Health Care, 12.

Chapter 16: Dry Cough

20 For a description of the Sanatorium in Hamilton, Canada and medical evacuation of Inuit with TB, see: Shawn Selway, *Nobody*

Here Will Harm You: Mass Medical Evacuation from the Eastern Arctic 1950–1965, (Hamilton: Wolsak & Wynn, 2016).

21 Hilary Lyons, Memo on Tuberculosis in Bumpe Chiefdom, Serabu Hospital, circa 1980.

22 Mary Maher, *Serabu Hospital—Centre for Nurse Training and Outreach to the Community: Annual Report 1980,* Serabu, Sierra Leone (1981).

23 *Serabu Hospital—Centre for Nurse Training and Outreach to the Community: Annual Report 1979,* Serabu, Sierra Leone (1980), 13.

Chapter 17: Traditional Birth Attendants

24 Belmont Williams and Fatu Yumkella, *The Evaluation of Traditional Birth Attendants' Training Programme and Performance in Sierra Leone.* Sierra Leone Government Ministry of Health (1982), 2.

25 Hilary Lyons, *Midwifery Notes for Serabu Hospital's Village Health Committee,* circa 1979.

Chapter 18: Breakdowns and Breakthroughs

26 These types of referral delays are described in the "three-delays" model in obstetric care".

Chapter 20: Research Plans

27 Williams, and Yumkella, *The Evaluation of Traditional Birth,* 8.

Chapter 27: Brief Interlude and Final Year in Sierra Leone

28 Nancy C. Edwards and Cathy H. Tompkins, "An Approach to International Education in Primary Health Care," *Nurse Educator* 13, no. 2 (1988): 31-36.

29 Nancy Edwards, Susan Smith, and Susan French (1989). "McMaster's Link with Pakistan," *The Canadian Nurse* (March 1989): 30-33.

Chapter 30: Unfinished Business

30 Nancy C. Edwards, "Traditional Birth Attendants in Sierra Leone: Key Providers of Maternal and Child Health Care in West Africa," *Western Journal of Nursing Research* 9, no. 3 (1987): 335-347.

31 Nancy C. Edwards, Nicholas J. Birkett, and Paul A. Sengeh. "Payment for Deliveries in Sierra Leone," *Bulletin of the World Health Organization* 67, no. 2 (1989): 163-169.

Chapter 32: A Reboot

32 Nancy Edwards, et al., "International Collaborative Workshops: A 6-year Partnership Between Canada and China," *Nurse Educator* 25, no. 2 (2000): 1-7.

33 Nancy Edwards, Dao Hui Zou, and Li Xi Song, "Continuing Education for Nurses in Tianjin Municipality, The People's Republic of China," *The Journal of Continuing Education in Nursing* 32, no. 1 (2001): 31-37.

34 University of Ottawa and Yunnan Provincial Public Health Bureau, *Sino-Canada Yunnan Maternal and Child Health Project (1997–2003): Final Report.* Submitted to Canadian International Development Agency, May 2003.

35 Nancy Edwards and Susan Roelofs, "Sustainability: The Elusive Dimension of International Health Projects," *Canadian Journal of Public Health* 97, no. 1 (2006): 45-49.

36 The countries involved in this project changed as indicated in the following communique: In 2007, a large multidisciplinary team of researchers and decision-makers from Canada and five LMICs (Barbados, Jamaica, Kenya, Uganda, and South Africa) received funding to implement a participatory action research programme entitled "Strengthening Nurses' Capacity for HIV Policy Development in Sub-Saharan Africa and the Caribbean." One year after programme funding was received and prior to any data collection, Barbados withdrew from the programme, with the four remaining partner countries continuing.

37 For project details, see: Nancy Edwards, et al., "The Impact of Leadership Hubs on the Uptake of Evidence-informed Nursing Practices and Workplace Policies for HIV Care: A Quasi-experimental Study in Jamaica, Kenya, Uganda, and South Africa," *Implementation Science* 11, 110 (2015). https://doi.org/10.1186/s13012-016-0478-3.

38 For project details, see: Charles Wafula, Nancy Edwards, and Daniel Kaseje, "Contextual Variations in Costs for a Community Health Strategy Implemented in Rural, Peri-urban, and Nomadic Sites in Kenya," *BMC Public Health*, 17, 224 (2017). https://doi.org/10.1186/s12889-017-4140-z.

39 For details, see: Nancy Edwards, Erica Di Ruggiero, and Sarah Viehbeck, "Chapter 15: Building the Field of Population Health Intervention Research Within a National Research Funding Agency," in *Developing a Program of Research: An Essential Process for a Successful Research Career*, ed. Nancy Edwards (Vancouver: CHNET Press, 2018), 325-351.

Chapter 33: Personal Reflections

40 For a discussion of the World Health Organization typology of FGM/C, see: Rigmor C. Berg, V. Odgaard-Jensen Underland, A. Fretherm, and G.E. Vist, "Effects of Female Genital Cutting on Physical Health Outcomes: A Systematic Review and Meta-analysis," *BMJ Open* 4 (2014). https://doi.org/10.1136/bmjopen-2014-006316.

41 For a discussion of FGM/C in historical context, see: Richard Fanthorpe, *Sierra Leone: The Influence of the Secret Societies, with Special Reference to Female Genital Mutilation*, Writenet Report, August 2007. https://www.refworld.org/pdfid/46cee3152.pdf.

42 For a discussion of FGM/C and Mende Secret Societies, see: Ngambouk Vitalis Pemunta, and Tabi Chama-James Tabenyang, "Cultural Power, Ritual Symbolism, and Human Rights Violations in Sierra Leone," *Cogent Social Sciences*, 3, no. 2 (2017). https://doi.org/10.1080/23311886.2017.1295549.

43 See for example: Dennis Kabatto, "Female Circumcision Awareness Week—Dr. Fuambai Sia Ahmadu Speaks," *The Sierra Leone Telegraph*, February 7, 2018. https://www.thesierraleonetelegraph.com/female-circumcision-awareness-week-dr-fuambai-sia-ahmadu-speaks/.

44 For a discussion of the Bondo Society and its hierarchy, see: Aisha Fofana Ibrahim. "The Bondo Society as a Political Tool: Examining Cultural Expertise in Sierra Leone from 1961 to 2018," *Laws* 8, no. 3 (2019). https://doi.org/10.3390/laws8030017.

45 See: UN Global Database on Violence Against Women, 2010–2013. Response of the Government of Sierra Leone to the Questionnaire on Violence Against Women (2010). https://evaw-global-database.unwomen.org/fr/countries/africa/sierra-leone/2010/national-gender-strategic-plan-2010-2013.

46 *The Agenda for Prosperity: Road to Middle Income Status. Sierra Leone's Third Generation. Poverty Reduction Strategy Paper (2013–2018),* Government of Sierra Leone. http://www.sierra-leone.org/Agenda%204%20Prosperity.pdf.

47 Abdul Rashid Thomas, "Bondo Leaders Vow to Uphold Government Policy on Protecting Girls," *The Sierra Leone Telegraph*, May 24, 2017. https://www.thesierraleonetelegraph.com/bondo-leaders-vow-to-uphold-government-policy-on-protecting-girls/.

48 Mathieu Maheu-Giroux et al., "Risk factors for Vaginal Fistula Symptoms in Sub-Saharan Africa: A pooled Analysis of National Household Survey Data," *BMC Pregnancy and Childbirth*, 16, 82 (2016). https://doi.org/10.1186/s12884-016-0871-6.

49 See: The Lomé Peace Agreement reached between the Government of Sierra Leone and the Revolutionary United Front of Sierra Leone. https://peaceaccords.nd.edu/wp-content/accords/The_Lome_Peace_Agreement-_1999_0.pdf.

50 Serabu Hospital was rebuilt and re-equipped by the organization German Doctors commencing in 2010.

51 Paul Sengeh and George Gage have provided leadership for a non-governmental, Sierra Leonean organization that focuses on the first 1,000 days of children's lives. See: https://focus1000.org/.

52 Dr. Belmont Williams has written about her experiences in Sierra Leone including the design of the Traditional Birth Attendant training program in *Right to Health: Women, Children and Culture*. (Del Sarto Publishing, 2020).

53 *National Ebola Recovery Strategy for Sierra Leone, 2015–2017*, Government of Sierra Leone, July 2015, 6. http://ebolaresponse. un.org/sites/default/files/sierra_leone_recovery_strategy_en.pdf.

54 Gianluca Quaglio et al., "Impact of Ebola Outbreak on Reproductive Health Services in a Rural District of Sierra Leone: A Prospective Observational Study," *BMJ Open*, 9 (2019). doi: 10.1136/bmjopen-2019-029093.

55 UNICEF, The Long-term Impacts and Costs of Ebola on the Sierra Leonean Health Sector (2019). https://www.unicef.org/ sierraleone/media/316/file/LTICESLHS-Report-2019.pdf.

CPSIA information can be obtained
at www.ICGtesting.com
Printed in the USA
LVHW040206200922
728808LV00003B/392